WRITE YOUR SKIN
A PRESCRIPTION FOR CHANGE

WRITE YOUR SKIN
A PRESCRIPTION FOR CHANGE

KATIE RODAN, MD
and
KATHY FIELDS, MD

with Lori Bush

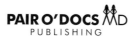

PAIR O' DOCS MD
PUBLISHING

Pair O' Docs Publishing San Francisco, CA

Published by
Pair O' Docs Publishing
60 Spear Street, Suite 600
San Francisco, CA 94105

Publisher's Cataloging-in-Publication Data
Rodan, Katie.

Prescription for change : write your skin a / Katie Rodan, Kathy Fields, with Lori Bush. – San Francisco, CA : Pair O' Docs Pub., 2010.

p. ; cm.

ISBN13: 978–0–9824608–0–1

1. Skin—Care and hygiene. 2. Face—Care and hygiene. I. Title.
II. Fields, Kathy, 1958- III. Bush, Lori.

RL87.R64 2010

646.726—dc22   2009903826

Project coordination assistance by Jenkins Group, Inc.
www.BookPublishing.com

FIRST EDITION, FIFTH PRINTING, 2014

Book design by Hint® Creative
Cover Photograph by Jeff Katz
Interior Photography by Jaime Fritsch, Derek Israelsen, and Robert Schlatter
Printed in the United States of America

16 15 14 13 • 7 6 5

Contents

Introduction: How Vanity Can Help You Go the Distance—Our Philosophy on Beauty, Skin, and Aging

Across cultures, men historically have looked for women with clear skin, high-arched eyebrows, full lips, and a cherubic face. These qualities, recognized as beautifully feminine, are the physical features associated with women at peak fertility. We've all heard it said that men look more distinguished as they age, that they become more masculine in appearance. The unfortunate reality is that women do, too. As women age, they, too, become more "handsome" because their skin and facial features begin to lose the defining characteristics that the human brain recognizes as feminine. Because of a decline in the feminizing hormones estrogen and progesterone, both men and women take on more traditionally male physical features with age. The face becomes angular as a result of fat loss, eyebrows flatten, facial hair grows, lips thin. While these traits can make a man look rugged or attractive, they tend to make a woman appear less feminine, more tired, and, overall, less desirable.

As we develop the wisdom of life experiences and the inner beauty that comes only with time and maturity, there remains a self-imposed critic that equates our self-worth with what is reflected in the bathroom mirror. While it is absolutely imperative that we adjust our expectations and redefine what is beautiful as we age, feeling good about the way we look is critical to our well-being. For many years, women believed they could do little or nothing about the state of their skin and the ravages of aging. Now, thankfully, it is possible to become an active participant in the quest for healthier, more attractive skin.

We want you to feel confident in your skin every day. That's why we wrote this book—to share our experiences and professional information about skin so you can make wise choices, whether at home or in the dermatologist's office, that will leave your skin looking its best. Looking good means feeling good, and it can be transformational; we see it every day.

> "Our patients are our inspiration. We've witnessed the transformation in confidence and self-esteem a person goes through as she gains control over frustrating skincare issues and knows her skin looks great. Our goal with this book is to extend our patient privilege to you by offering the best skincare solutions straight from our offices. We want all people to experience their best skin; it's easier than you may think."
>
> **DR. KATIE RODAN** and
> **DR. KATHY FIELDS**

Your Skin Is Your Best Marketing Tool

Because clear, radiant skin is a natural outcome of health and well-being, a luminous, even-toned, unblemished complexion is universally recognized as beautiful and is a very precious asset. And this, in theory, is how nature intended it to be. According to Nina Jablonski, anthropologist and author of *Skin: A Natural History*, "Our skin reflects our ... state of health ... and much of what we want the world to know about us."[2] Human beings are programmed to be attracted to individuals who best reflect inner health through outer beauty.

The quest for perfectly smooth, flawless, soft, supple skin is nothing new. Noted British zoologist Desmond Morris claims that, evolutionarily, the most universally desirable and attractive feature among humans is not flowing blonde hair, abundant breasts, or long legs but perfect, clear skin.[3] In fact, 40,000 years ago a cavewoman with unsightly skin problems would have been seen as diseased and banished from her tribe. Today, if your skin doesn't look good, you may feel as much an outsider as our ancestors did.

But 40,000 years ago our purpose was simply to procreate, raise our children until they reached maturity, and then die so as not to use the resources needed for the younger generation. Up until the turn of the nineteenth century, our life expectancy was around only forty-six years, so there was no purpose in worrying about how we aged. Today, however, we may easily live well into our eighties or nineties. Even with nature and hormones working against us, our appearance remains a critical aspect of our self-esteem. We need our skin to last and look good as long as we do.

Starting at a young age, our skin becomes our best—or worst—marketing tool. When we reach puberty, we start to become aware of our bodies and our sexuality. Subconsciously, the search for a mate begins. It is also at this critical time in development that we feel the most insecure and vulnerable. Hormones play a cruel twist of fate as they unleash troubled skin with acne and dandruff. Unwanted breakouts, at a time when one's peers are truly looking, can derail self-esteem and affect confidence for the rest of our lives.

Whether you're eighteen or eighty-one, the desire to be desirable never goes away. The issues may change from acne to wrinkles, but the requirement to look good remains. That's why we maintain that "vanity" is not a dirty word.

It's not vain to want to look as good as you feel. In fact, we are giving you permission to be vain. It can be a positive thing. It means looking after yourself and striving to be the best you can be. When you stop caring about how you look, it's a sign of giving up. If everyone around you is saying "You look tired" and you're just really tired of hearing it, it's time to take action.

Natural Beauty

We are big believers in real, natural beauty. It's not about having perfect features; it's about rejuvenation without distortion. Artificial beauty doesn't count. It's amazing how much you can do for yourself at home by combining topical treatments with healthy habits and the occasional in-office dermatological procedure. Although it's tempting, don't use celebrities and models as your benchmark of beauty. You don't have a professional makeup artist following you around, and you can't airbrush your face. Hollywood just isn't reality.

The Obstacles to Getting Great Skin

As practicing dermatologists with more than forty years of combined clinical experience, we treat hundreds of skin conditions. We've witnessed firsthand the emotional scars that acne and other common concerns such as wrinkles, hyperpigmentation, and skin sensitivity can cause. We've also observed the confusion and frustration women have about how best to care for their skin. Most of the time, they just don't know where to turn for advice.

That's not surprising. With fewer than ten thousand dermatologists in the United States treating a population of more than three hundred million, it's easy to see why most people have never seen a dermatologist. In fact, we often become the most popular women at cocktail parties. People seek us out to ask those "Oh, by the way" questions they don't ask their doctors. When it comes to your skin and seeking medical attention, no question should be too embarrassing or too vain. We've diagnosed melanoma on patients who came in to get a Botox treatment. We also know there are numerous skin conditions that may not be pressing enough for you to see a dermatologist about, and we'll give you the knowledge to self-treat many of these concerns.

Knowledge Is Power and Beauty— Be Your Own Dermatologist

Because the journey to great skin can be fraught with confusion and a consultation with a dermatologist may be unrealistic, we want to empower you to become your own dermatologist of sorts. After all, a little knowledge is a beautiful thing. We want to help you understand your skin well enough to make smart, logical decisions and stamp out confusion by separating the scientifically sound treatments and products from all the wannabes. We want to teach you how to look at your face the way we do by educating you about your skin and giving you inside access to what happens behind the closed doors of the dermatologist's office.

To that end, we've created this book as your "bedside dermatologist"—a comprehensive and hopefully entertaining go-to guide containing all the information you need to successfully care for your skin, hair, and nails. We have enlisted the help of skincare industry veteran Lori Bush to help make our dermatology-speak reader friendly. If you're wondering why you have acne at forty, how to treat that red, sensitive patch on your cheek, or what the latest procedure is to get rid of a wrinkle, you have a source for the information and a place to come back to time and again.

Your take-home message from the chapters that follow is that you have choices. The choices you make today will affect the way you look and feel tomorrow, next year, and well into the future. You can start by replacing bad daily habits with good ones. Our interactive exercises can help you follow our suggested programs for reversing much of the damage that already has been done to restore a healthy, clear, even-toned complexion. And you can take steps to protect your skin from the sun and environment to prevent future damage from surfacing. With this book, you literally can write your own prescription for change.

> "I have a beautiful, professional fifty-year-old patient who is armed with magazine articles and advertisements every time she comes in for a treatment. She says 'I see all these ads and everything sounds great, but I'm skeptical that any of it will work. I have no idea what to do with my skin. Please help me!' Our goal is to clear up the confusion so you can make smart decisions for the sake of your skin.
>
> **DR. KATIE RODAN**

A Prescription for Change—You Control Your Skin's Destiny

Instead of reading palms, we read the back of your hands. Skin can expose your history of healthy or unhealthy lifestyles choices. If your skin has been protected from the environment, it will look youthful well beyond its years. On the other hand, even moderate levels of environmental stress such as unprotected sun exposure tremendously accelerate the skin's aging process, producing a sallow, mottled, ruddy, and wrinkled complexion.

In the chapters that follow, we will address everything from the physiology and aging of skin to the impact of hormones and the sun. You have control over 80% of how your skin will age. We will let you know how to control and combat the key aging culprits. We will also discuss treatments for common dermatologic problems. We'll include case studies, excerpts from journal articles, surveys, list, charts, and lots of great information to educate, entertain, and empower you. When medical procedures are a valuable option, we'll walk you through technology and product alternatives, highlighting which ones provide the greatest benefits so that you can make informed decisions. We'll give you our insider tips and introduce you to the best of what is available. Finally, we'll help you develop a checklist of questions to bring with you should you decide a visit to your dermatologist is in order.

We want to offer you what we give to our patients every day—sound advice and counsel about your skin. It's almost like bringing the dermatologist to your home and is our idea of the modern house call. We're offering you a common sense, logical approach so you can make a lifestyle commitment to healthy, beautiful skin. And remember: it's never too late to change your skin's destiny.

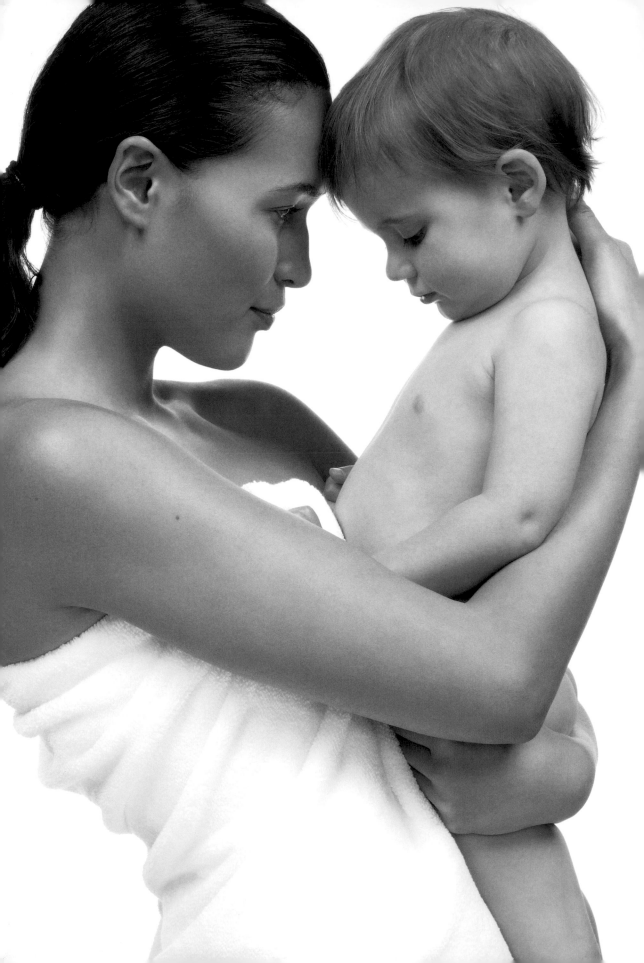

YOUR SKIN'S DESTINY

What's in Store?

"There is no cure for the common birthday."

Astronaut and Senator John Glenn

Genetics are pretty amazing. Most of us take great delight in observing how the same DNA manifests itself differently among family members, making for great people watching at a mall. As women, we often benchmark our mothers to get a sense of how we might look in twenty or thirty years. And we know that our boyfriends scrutinize our moms' appearances for the same reason.

But as times change, our familial elders are providing a less predictive crystal ball into our future faces. That's because science has taught us that DNA accounts for only 20% of visible aging changes. Our environment and our daily habits are responsible for a whopping 80%. And that's great news! You, not your parents, are in the driver's seat ultimately controlling your skin's destiny.

With advances in skincare technology, even if you thought you were a goner as a result of years of abuse to your body, all is not lost. You can start today on your road to skin rehab, implementing corrective measures and substituting newfound good habits for the old bad ones.

It's never too late to be proactive. Discover how, by incorporating the right skincare choices into your daily personal care routine, your skin can literally improve with age, allowing you to look better tomorrow than you did yesterday.

The earlier you start, the better. With any skin condition, the old adage "An ounce of prevention is worth a pound of cure" holds true. We proved with Proactiv® Solution that treating acne-prone skin prevents pimples from appearing. Similarly, it's best to prevent sun damage before the dullness appears and treat your skin for aging before a wrinkle forms.

Skin: More Than Just Window Dressing

Before we get into the details of aging and how you can prevent the dreaded signs, let's take a step back and talk a little bit about skin in general.

As dermatologists, we have developed a profound respect and appreciation for skin as an organ. But beyond the critical role it plays in your appearance, skin possesses many impressive features and functions that have adapted and evolved in ways essential to the sustainability of the human species.

Skin Anatomy and Physiology Primer (As Painless As We Can Make It)

One of the most important things you can do to ensure your health and longevity, whether it relates to skin or any other biological system, is to be an active participant. Spending a few minutes now learning about the three layers of your skin will give you insight that will serve your skin well for years into the future.

The View from the Top: The Epidermis

The top layer of skin is called the epidermis, and the very top layer of the epidermis is called the stratum corneum, or barrier layer. Although the stratum corneum is composed entirely of dead skin cells, it performs a highly critical role in our overall health. It retains moisture for our living tissue and virtually prohibits the entry of germs and most chemicals into our bodies.

The epidermis consists of several living layers below the stratum corneum and is made up of three different cell types—keratinocytes, melanocytes, and Langerhans cells. All three cell types play an important role in the health and appearance of skin.

Keratinocytes: Keeping Them Turning

Comprising the majority of the epidermis, keratinocytes provide structure to the skin, hair, and nails. Below the barrier layer, keratinocytes are metabolically active cells, responding to stimuli from the environment to regulate proliferation and development of other cells in the skin.

New keratinocytes are born at the base of the epidermis. As they mature, they travel up to the skin's surface, morphing along the way into dry, flat discs called horn cells, or corneocytes. At the skin's surface, their new flat shape allows them to lie on top of each other, like shingles on a roof, to form the stratum corneum.

Eventually, the stratum corneum cells simply flake off one by one and become the primary source of house dust (icky but true). In a young person, the keratinocyte maturation process, from start to dust, takes twenty-eight to thirty days, except in certain skin conditions where the process speeds up, but more on that later. This means the epidermis completely renews itself every month. That's why young skin always looks so fresh and rosy.

Problematically, the process of epidermal renewal slows as you age, so much so that by the time you're forty, it could take fifty days or more for the skin to rejuvenate. When dead cells don't slough off as rapidly, your stratum corneum gets thicker, appearing almost stale, and the dead cells pack into your pores, making them look larger. Beautiful skin is determined by light reflectance. A thicker layer of dead skin cells lying on the surface of your face gives you a sallow and dull appearance. This is why exfoliation becomes increasingly important. It assists the natural shedding process and reveals the newer, fresher skin cells below.

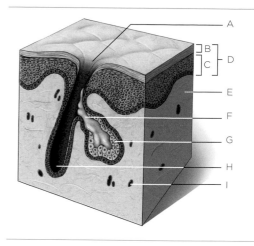

A: Pore
B: Stratum corneum
C: Keratinocytes, melanocytes, Langerhans
D: Epidermis
E: Dermis, contains collagen and elastin
F: Sebum (oil)
G: Sebaceous (oil) gland
H: Empty hair follicle
I: Blood vessels

Why Did the Apartment Get So Dusty?

"I recently conducted a de facto experiment of keratinocyte shedding. Three friends came to stay with me for a long weekend in my San Francisco flat. Whereas I normally need to dust only every couple of weeks (I'm not there much), the place was literally coated in dust by the time they left. They shed their dead skin cells all over the place!" *Lori Bush*

The epidermis, the outermost layer of skin, sheds a million dead cells every forty minutes. That adds up to 1.5 pounds a year. By the time you reach age seventy, a whopping 105 pounds will have been lost—and that's without a diet! Unlike a snake that completely sheds its skin every year, humans do it on a continuous basis, creating more than one thousand brand-new skins in a lifetime. These dead skin cells constitute more than 90% of house dust.

Melanocytes: Few in Number, Big on Impact

Melanocytes are cells that produce melanin, the pigment that gives skin its color. Although melanocytes account for only 5%–10% of our epidermal cells, their impact on our appearance is profound and often unpredictable.

As we age, we observe changes in the number and productivity of our melanocytes. We naturally lose melanocytes, thus diminishing the pigment-producing capacity of our skin. Our skin becomes lighter and less protected and sunburns more easily than it did in our youth. But these changes vary significantly from individual to individual and depend greatly on how we care for our skin.

Sun exposure has the most profound effect on melanocytes. From our very first day at the park, ultraviolet radiation causes melanocytes to become enlarged and overactive, particularly in fairer-skinned individuals. Over time, this increased melanocyte activity causes the formation of brown spots, which we refer to as freckles in children and liver spots in the elderly. At the same time, chronic sun exposure may lead to total depigmentation due to destruction of melanocytes. The evidence of this is the appearance of white dots scattered most prominently on the forearm and chin. We'll discuss the effects of sun damage on skin pigmentation in more detail in Chapter Nine.

Langerhans Cells: Protection from Infection

When infectious microbes manage to work their way through the skin's protective barrier, Langerhans cells are mobilized, triggering the production of antibodies, which respond to the invasion of this foreign DNA. Thus, despite being the most exposed organ of our body, skin is surprisingly resistant to infection. Unfortunately, Langerhans cell numbers diminish with age, weakening the skin's immunity to fight both infection and skin cancer.

The Dermis: Where We Get Collagen and Elastin

The middle layer of skin is made up of sebaceous (oil) glands, sweat glands, hair follicles, fibroblasts, and the two important structural proteins they produce: collagen and elastin. Collagen gives skin its strength and fullness, while elastin gives skin its elasticity and stretch.

Both collagen and elastin naturally diminish or break down with age and chronic sun exposure. As these supportive fibers deplete, the skin becomes thinner overall, capillaries become more apparent, skin tears or bruises easily, and wounds heal more slowly. Additionally, pores become enlarged when collagen and elastin fibers collapse. As if that weren't enough, the smooth, taut skin of youth becomes wrinkled and loose.

Blood vessels are made up of collagen and cushioned by surrounding fat cells. The breakdown of collagen and disappearance of fat that comes gradually with age cause our vessels to become fragile and leaky. By your fifties, you may notice that minimal trauma produces large, dark purple bruises on your extremities that seem to last for weeks. On your face and chest, the loss of collagen causes tiny capillaries to expand, and sun damage further promotes the growth of new blood vessels. This results in a diffuse redness on the cheeks, neck, and chest. Enlarged red capillaries, often referred to as "broken blood vessels," become prominent fixtures around the nose.

How Collagen and Elastin Change with Location and Age

The amount of collagen and elastin in the dermal layer of skin varies in different parts of the body. You can easily do a personal demonstration to prove how the strength and stretch of the skin varies on different parts of your own body. Take your finger and gently pull the delicate skin under your eye and then pull the skin on your thigh. Notice how much thicker and more taut the skin on the thigh is compared with that of the eye area. No wonder the eyes are often the first place to show the signs of aging.

Now, test changes associated with age. With your index finger and thumb, pinch the skin on the back of your hand. How quickly does it snap back into place? Try this on somebody who is much younger or much older than you and note the difference in how far the skin comes up and the rate at which it returns when you let go.

Collagen and Wound Repair: The Birth of a Scar

The dermal layer is also where collagen is produced in response to an injury. When injury occurs, nature works as quickly as possible to fill the void. In the process, bundles of disorganized collagen are often produced, and in the body's overzealous attempt to heal, it creates far more collagen than is necessary. Disorganized and excessive collagen creates scars, which may look like pits, dents, or ropey thickenings. You may have heard of keloids; these are pink, firm, elevated scars especially common in African Americans. Because keloids extend well beyond the borders of the injury, something as small as an ear piercing can leave a huge disfiguring keloidal-type scar. Unfortunately, once a scar, always a scar. However, cosmetic dermatology has means of camouflaging or modifying scars, which we will share with you later.

The Subcutaneous Layer: Where Fat Is Beautiful

The bottom layer of skin consists of fat cells and deeper hair follicles. Fat gives skin its full, firm cushion and softness. We admire it in youth. In fact, it's the reason we all love to kiss a baby's fat cheek. However, our national obsession with weight loss has us believing that as we age, all fat is bad. As dermatologists, we know that a little fat in just the right places can be a good thing. Yet, with aging, we tend to naturally lose our facial fat pad. Hollows replace the round contours of youthful cheeks, giving us a tired, gaunt appearance. That's why the French have the saying "It's either your face or your fanny."

Because cosmetic surgery doesn't repair fat loss, dermatologists use techniques to inject the face with fillers, restoring some fullness to give the face a younger, more lifted look. Admittedly, however, even the best of the new fillers can't return a certain youthful glow. That's because our original fat releases hormones and stores estrogen, greatly enhancing the youthful appearance of skin.

"If you bought a car and knew it had to last you for a hundred years, wouldn't you take care of it differently than if you thought it could be replaced? Wouldn't you check out every rattle and fix every ding? Wouldn't you fill it with high-octane fuel? I bet you'd do anything to take care of that car if you knew it had to last a lifetime. Most of us don't do that for our bodies. But if we did, we'd look and feel a lot better."

DR. KATIE RODAN

You can really see the impact of fat depletion in celebrity photos. Look at actresses who were popular in their twenties such as Michelle Pfeiffer and Demi Moore. Their faces were round and full. In their thirties and forties, the fat layer started to deplete, making them look lean, sculpted, and more defined. But as the fat layer continues to thin, the eventual result is a gaunt, tired, aged appearance.

Does Skin Tone Affect Aging?

If you think everyone ages at the same rate, think again. The color of your skin contributes not only to your individual uniqueness but also to the way in which your skin reacts to the environment and how quickly it ages. In general, the darker your complexion, the better able your skin is to resist environmental assaults and the more slowly it ages, but all skin tones are negatively impacted by the sun to a greater or lesser extent. For example, if you are a fifty-year-old fair-complected woman who religiously protected herself from the sun, your skin will appear to age more slowly compared with that of your sun-worshipping peers, regardless of their ethnicities.

How Different Skin Tones Age

ADVANTAGES OF DARK- AND MEDIUM-TONED SKIN:	DISADVANTAGES OF DARK- AND MEDIUM-TONED SKIN:
Skin tone helps hide redness, which is a feature of many skin conditions from rosacea to broken capillaries Darker complexions often have larger fat cushions beneath the skin, keeping the face fuller and less wrinkled	Denser population of melanocytes produces more uneven discoloration with sun exposure Following trauma, more prone to dark marks (post-inflammatory hyperpigmentation), which can take months to years to fade Dead skin cells on the surface are more visible, often creating an "ashy" appearance A tendency to develop ingrown hairs and razor bumps called *Pseudofolliculitis barbae*, especially in those with curly hair More prone to keloid scars

ADVANTAGES OF LIGHT-TONED SKIN:	DISADVANTAGES OF LIGHT-TONED SKIN:
Not as prone to the development of dark marks following trauma (post-inflammatory hyperpigmentation) More responsive to lightening treatments, including lasers and topical lighteners such as hydroquinone Less tendency to heal with a visible keloid-type scar Better response to laser hair removal	Extremely prone to sunburn Greater tendency to wrinkle from environmental exposure More prone to facial redness and "broken capillaries" stemming from conditions such as rosacea Thinner fat layer producing a more gaunt appearance with aging

Nature versus Nurture

Skin ages in two ways: intrinsically and extrinsically. Intrinsic, biologic aging includes factors such as genetics, ethnicity, and one's underlying health or disease state. We call it the "who you are" component of aging. However, as mentioned earlier, intrinsic aging accounts for only 20% or so of the visible aging process, much of which is under your control. So, even if you didn't inherit a fabulous complexion, great skin has more to do with what you do to it than with what you've been given.

Top Extrinsic Aging Factors

- Sunlight
- Smoking
- Amount of sleep and sleep positions
- Stress
- Diet and dieting

- Exercise
- Climate
- Alcohol
- Facial expressions

We'll let you know how you can take control of each extrinsic factor in Chapter Two.

On the other hand, extrinsic, environmental aging accounts for 80% of your appearance and is greatly under your control. It includes factors such as sun exposure, smoking, excessive alcohol intake, and diet. We call that the "what you do" element of aging.

Twin Studies and Why We Love Them

Studies of identical twins demonstrate the clear difference between nature and nurture, or the effects of genetics versus lifestyle. In 2008, researchers from King's College London published a study in the *Archives of Internal Medicine* based upon observation of 2,401 pairs of identical twins. They discovered that a sedentary lifestyle plays a major role in the aging process. Extracting DNA samples from volunteers, they found that those who vigorously exercised three hours a week had longer telomeres and were biologically nine years younger than those who exercised fewer than fifteen minutes weekly. (Telomeres are found at the end of a chromosome, protecting the DNA and enabling cells to replicate. With each cellular replication, telomeres shorten, eventually becoming so small that cell replication is impossible, causing cellular death.) Their research was adjusted for body weight, smoking, economic status, and physical activity at work. Amazingly, even one and a half hours of exercise per week reduced biological age by four years.[1]

Because identical twins share the same genetic makeup, it was previously believed they would age in exactly the same way. This study demonstrated that a twin enjoying a lifestyle of regular exercise, minimal sun exposure, a healthy diet, limited alcohol consumption, and no smoking aged noticeably better than her twin who made poorer lifestyle choices. The study also proved that she would not only look better but also outlive her sister.

Your Skin's Future

Sound depressing? It's really not as bad as you may think. In this chapter we've offered basic information on aging skin to empower you to positively affect the outcome. There is so much you can do today to improve your health and skin tomorrow. In other words, you can reverse many of the most common signs of aging and take control of your skin. All it takes is the right attitude and, of course, a combination of products, ingredients, treatments, and lifestyle changes.

Top Ten Signs Your Skin Is Getting Old

1. Your stratum corneum (the very top layer of the skin) becomes thicker, making skin look dull, flaky, and less radiant.

2. Fine lines and wrinkles become more pronounced.

3. As natural exfoliation slows, pores become clogged with dead skin cells and appear larger and stretched out.

4. Skin becomes thinner and less firm as collagen breaks down and decreases in production.

5. Melanocyte production decreases, which results in skin pallor and uneven tone.

6. With the decrease in production of Langerhans cells, the skin's immune system is compromised. Therefore, wounds heal more slowly, and skin cancers may occur more often.

7. Skin becomes dryer as sebaceous glands grow larger but produce less oil.

8. Broken and dilated capillaries appear on skin as a result of a lifetime of sun exposure.

9. Uneven skin tone in the form of dark spots or hyperpigmentation increases, again because of the sun.

10. Skin bruises more easily as blood vessels weaken.

✏ Write Your Prescription for Change

Your personal prescription for change starts with identifying your most pressing skin problems. In medicine, we call it triaging—prioritizing issues in order to treat the most urgent problem first. So, let's get started.

STEP 1: Stand in front of the mirror.

STEP 2: Think of everything you would like to improve, such as:
- acne or breakouts
- brown spots or uneven skin tone
- dull, drab skin
- large pores
- fine lines, wrinkles
- sagging skin
- facial redness

STEP 3: Write them in their order of importance to you.

1. _____

2. _____

3. _____

4. _____

In the chapters that follow, we will cover the items on your list. You might want to bookmark this page so you can easily refer to it.

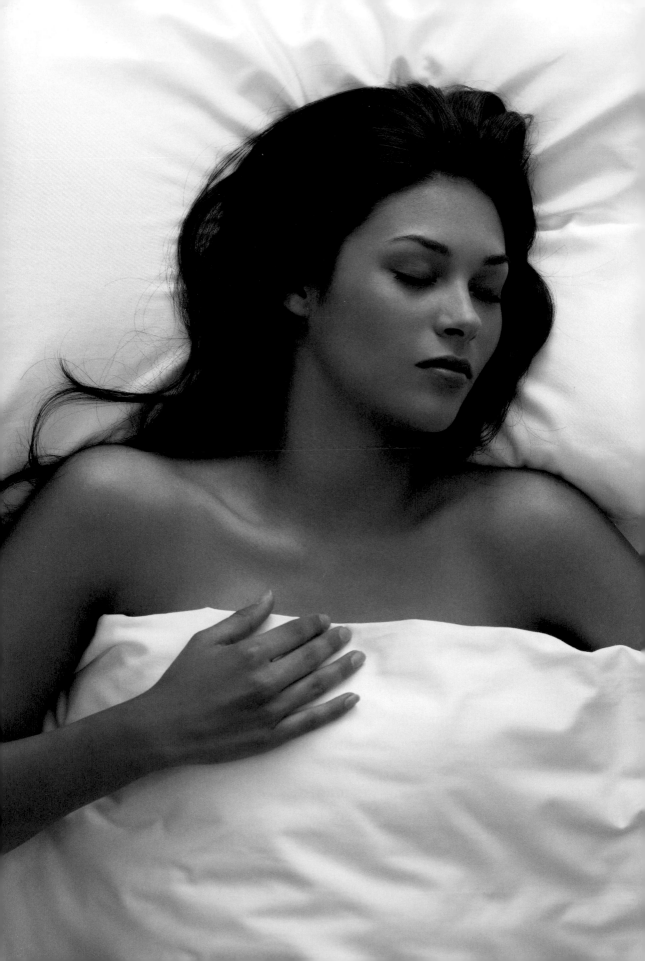

SKINCARE TRUTHS AND MYTHS

What to Do, What to Skip

"Back in the early '70s, my best friend's mom, a former Miss California, taught me her beauty secret for cleansing. Start by steaming your face with very hot water to open the pores, and then after washing, immediately dip your face in ice water to close them. It took me until my dermatology residency to learn that pores don't have the equivalent of mini-mouths."

Dr. Katie Rodan

There's a lot of confusion out there. People are bombarded with contradicting skincare information and a cluttered marketplace. To help you discern fact from fiction and clear up the confusion, we're offering advice straight from our dermatology practices. We're devoting this entire chapter to healthy habits you should implement as well as "skin myths" you should just plain ignore.

Madison Avenue images, from tanned, über-thin models to drug-addicted, cigarette-smoking superstars, create an illusion that a risky lifestyle is sexy and powerful. These images seem to be saying, "Look at all the things I can do to myself and still look great."

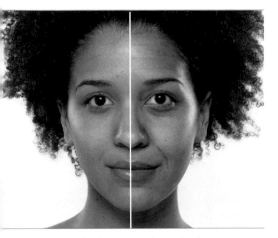

Natural aging vs. accelerated aging

Subconsciously, the ability of one's body to survive such bad habits and look beautiful in the process is perceived as a testament of strength and fertility. Promoting the benefits of a healthy diet, sun protection, and not smoking to those who possess the beauty and sense of invincibility of youth is often impossible. However, as we tell our patients every day, many of the skincare battles that are faced later in life are more easily prevented than they are corrected.

While aging is inevitable, your daily behaviors and choices greatly influence how you look at each birthday. With that in mind, we've developed the following list of "Top Ten Healthy Skin Habits." If your lifestyle already includes these choices, congratulations—we're sure it shows. If, like many of us, your habits aren't quite up to par, now is the time to become more proactive in your skin's health and future.

Top Ten Healthy Skin Habits

1. PROTECT YOUR SKIN FROM THE SUN

Your skin is a terrific historian. It carries with it souvenirs of past vacations at the beach, pregnancies, picked pimples, and more. Many of the lasting undesirable changes that occur have a common ingredient in the mix: the sun.

It's easy to see what the sun has done to your skin over time. Compare the skin on the inside of your arm with that on the outside of your arm and on the back of your hands. If you're like most people, the skin on the inside is smooth, clear, firm, and unmarked, while the skin on the outside is "dry roasted": freckled, dry, finely lined, not as firm, and possibly dotted with brown spots. And if you spend much time driving (in the United States), your left arm is probably worse than your right. Skin is simply closer to perfection "where the sun don't shine." And those are just the cosmetic effects. For the full scoop on how sun affects your skin, refer to Chapter Five.

Years of advertising have taught us to love the look of a tan. Let's set the record straight, and there is no bending this rule: there is no such thing as a healthy tan. Sun exposure damages skin, and the

Dead Giveaway

Madeleine is a young model who smoked to stay thin. We explained to her the risk of cancer associated with smoking, but she wasn't interested in quitting until we told her that eventually her looks would suffer and her career would be at risk. That did it. Madeleine flipped out and quit. We appreciate how addictive smoking is, but whatever it takes to quit, be it fear or vanity, it's worth it.

We can always tell whether a patient is a smoker. She looks about ten years older than her chronological age: her teeth are yellow, and her face is gaunt, sallow, and covered with fine lines and deep wrinkles. And this isn't just in older women. In fact, we've witnessed the characteristic "smoker's face" in women as young as thirty-five.

pigment you see as a tan is the body's reaction to this injury. There's nothing "healthy" or pretty about damaged skin.

The most important thing you can do to keep your skin looking young, not to mention healthy, is never to expose unprotected skin to the sun. Slather your skin with a broad-spectrum UVA/UVB sunscreen and apply it often. It's the ultimate wrinkle cream.

2. DON'T SMOKE—EVER!

Smoking literally affects the structure of the skin. Into the body by way of the bloodstream, smoking delivers thousands of toxins including carbon monoxide, nicotine, formaldehyde, lead, mercury, and tar. It causes skin's blood vessels to constrict, impairing circulation and the delivery of oxygen to skin tissue. It reduces skin's ability to form collagen and causes elastin to thicken and break apart. Smoking generates a tremendous number of free radicals while simultaneously interfering with the skin's ability to protect itself from free radicals. Smoking has also been shown to reduce the production of estrogen in women. The result: dryness, cracking, wrinkles, and sagging skin.

On top of that, the squinting and puckering associated with inhaling have been proven to increase wrinkling around the eyes and lips. A 1996 study headed by John Zone, MD, chairman of the University of Utah Department of Dermatology, measured the wrinkles in the faces of nonsmokers and smokers, establishing statistically and clinically that smokers' faces show more wrinkling at an earlier age than those of nonsmokers.[1]

Skin just plain doesn't work right when addicted to cigarettes: not only does smoking delay wound healing but also smokers are two to three times as likely to develop psoriasis as nonsmokers. Most alarmingly, research has shown a link between cigarette smoking and squamous cell cancer of the lips, as well as an increased death rate from melanoma.

Scientists at the Twin Research Unit at St. Thomas's Hospital in London looked at twenty-five pairs of identical twins where one was a lifelong smoker and the other had never smoked. Not only were the smokers more wrinkled but also the skin on the inside of their arms was up to 40% thinner than that of their nonsmoking siblings.[2]

With all this scientific evidence, it's obvious that smoking, like sun exposure, is nonnegotiable. If you are having difficulty quitting, we strongly recommend seeing your doctor for help.

Beneficial Pop Culture

"Wear sunscreen. If I could offer you only one tip for the future, sunscreen would be it. The long-term benefits of sunscreen have been proved by scientists, whereas the rest of my advice has no basis more reliable than my own meandering experience. I will dispense this advice now." Mary Schmich, *Chicago Tribune*, June 1, 1997[3]

This is one urban legend we actually like! The column written by Mary Schmich became a hoax and then a song when it was attributed to Kurt Vonnegut Jr. as an M.I.T. graduation speech.

3. GET YOUR BEAUTY SLEEP—ON YOUR BACK

Have you ever awakened in the morning and dragged yourself to the bathroom only to glance in the mirror and realize that you look like your passport photo?

If this happens more often than you'd like, the simple cause may be lack of sleep. Research has shown that most adults function best with eight to nine hours of sleep a night. However, a survey by the National Sleep Foundation found that 40% of adults get fewer than seven hours each night.[4] Whether because of your habit of burning the candle at both ends or biological disruptions of normal sleep patterns, this sleep deficit quickly takes a toll on you emotionally and physically, and your face is no exception.

We're all too familiar with the look. Dark circles show up under your eyes, and your complexion looks dull and gray. When your body is tired, skin pales, so the bluish blood vessels near the surface become more pronounced. Additionally, blood may seep from the tiny capillaries around the eyes, resulting in permanent dark shadows. Lack of sleep also raises cortisol and glucose levels, causing health problems such as hypertension and Type II diabetes, which in turn speed up the aging process.

Skin "rests" at night. When you sleep, the cells undergo repair and turn over slightly faster, helping your face look bright and refreshed. Therefore, if you don't get enough sleep, you won't look your best.

Just as important as getting a good night's sleep is the position in which you sleep. In 1987, Dr. Samuel J. Stegman first described "sleep creases"—the facial lines often mistaken for wrinkles that appear when you get up in the morning and deepen and persist over time. [5]

> "I never thought I could learn to sleep on my back, but with the help of a special pillow and a nightly pep talk, I've changed a lifelong habit. My reward—after a few weeks, my sleep crush lines disappeared like a newly ironed sheet."
>
> **DR. KATIE RODAN**

If you sleep facedown on a pillow or primarily on one side, the weight of your body and compression from the bedding will cause the creases. We call these diagonal lines across the forehead, from the lower eyelid to the bottom of the nose and through the lip and chin, "sleep crush."

In addition to the formation of these specific lines, your sleep position can also deepen the natural lines of facial expression. This is especially apparent in the nasolabial folds (the lines that connect the nostrils to the outer corners of the mouth) and the marionette lines that extend from the lower lip to the chin. We can often tell in what position a patient sleeps by the depth and location of facial lines.

How do you know whether a wrinkle is sleep crush? If it's diagonal and reversible with a change in sleep position, then it's sleep crush.

In Chapters Thirteen and Fifteen, we'll share various treatments that can help to diminish the appearance of lines that have been imprinted onto skin from years of sleeping position habits. But here's a piece of advice you can put into effect tonight and immediately share with others: train yourself to get off your side and sleep on your back. For lifelong side or facedown sleepers, this may feel uncomfortable at first, but you will get used to it. If you just can't train yourself to stay on your back through the night, try the Therapeutica Sleeping Pillow, which is specially contoured to support the head and cradle the neck. We've had patients who have noticed fewer wrinkles after using this special pillow for only a week.

Morning eyelid puffiness is another good reason to get into the habit of sleeping on your back. Sleeping position can lead to lymphedema or fluid retention in the tissue around the eyes, particularly if you are prone to these conditions. As skin ages and becomes slack, puffiness becomes even

Research at Stanford University's School of Medicine shows there may be a strong correlation between exam-related stress and acne severity in college students. A volunteer sample of students with varying degrees of acne was assessed during both nonexamination and examination periods. The result was that as students approached exams and experienced a higher level of stress, they also experienced more severe acne.[6] And according to an article from *Dermatology Insights,* 91% of respondents said that emotional stress caused or sometimes caused their rosacea flare-ups.[7]

more pronounced. Sleeping on your back, particularly propped up with your head raised above your heart, can help alleviate these under-eye bags.

Understand, too, that diet may contribute to puffy eyelids. So if you find yourself waking up with that not-so-bright-eyed look, try eliminating salty foods, caffeine, and alcohol from your diet, as they can cause water retention as well as interfere with sleep cycles.

If you do all the right things and still find yourself waking up puffy, placing ice packs on your eyelids or gently massaging the area can help. During the day, gravity will work in your favor, reducing the water retention around the eyes.

Getting your beauty rest really is important for your skin. So now that you're sleeping on your back, try these additional techniques for a better night's sleep:

- *Make a schedule and stick to it. Set your alarm for the same time each morning and get up when it goes off, even if you've gone to bed late the night before.*

- *Create a calm, comfortable environment that evokes rest: eliminate television, earphones, light. Some neurologists even believe the LED light from your alarm clock can lead to a less-than-optimal night's sleep and advise you to turn the clock away from your bed.*

- *Keep your bedroom cool.*

- *Stay away from coffee and alcohol four to six hours before bedtime.*

- *Don't go to bed with your stomach hungry or too full.*

- *Incorporate exercise into your daily routine.*

- *Keep a pad near your bed. When you wake up with your to-do list floating through your brain, write it down and go back to sleep.*

4. DON'T STRESS OUT

When our bodies are responding to stress, blood, nutrients, and oxygen are directed to the vital areas such as our legs and away from the nonvital organs such as the skin. The signs are obvious: an ashen or sallow appearance, flushed cheeks, dark under-eye circles, dull and limp hair, and more pronounced lines and wrinkles. Studies have shown that stress-induced cortisol inhibits the body's repair processes, decreases the rate of wound healing, increases the risk of infection, and triggers conditions such as acne, hives, eczema, psoriasis, rosacea, warts, and herpes. It can even bring on illnesses such as cancer and autoimmune disease. Recent research has shown that stress can cause telomeres to shorten and cells to die faster, effectively speeding up the aging process (see Chapter One).

Today we seem to live in a constant state of internal and external stress. In fact, psychologists estimate that the amount of stress an average adult undergoes in one day surpasses the amount of stress our cave-dwelling ancestors experienced in an entire year.

And You Thought Your Job Was Stressful...

As President Barack Obama embarked on the first months of his presidency, many alerted him to the theories of Dr. Michael Roizen, Cleveland Clinic's chief wellness officer. Dr. Roizen's studies suggest that the pressures on the commander-in-chief take measurable tolls on health and appearance and that the typical U.S. president ages two years for every year he is in office.[8] Have you ever compared pictures of Bill Clinton at the start of his presidency with those later into his term? He entered the presidency with salt-and-pepper hair and a twinkle in his eye but left with wrinkles and powder-white hair, appearing to have aged many years more than the eight he served.

The human species produces an excess amount of the hormone cortisol when under stress. In primitive times, the cortisol burst was necessary for the fight-or-flight response. However, while modern times rarely give us cause to physically escape an attacking savage beast, we are constantly faced with emotional stress that similarly causes a spike in cortisol. And when there is extra cortisol in our bodies that is not being used, the results can be quite destructive.

Maybe you were unexpectedly served with divorce papers, someone close to you died, or your company suddenly went bankrupt. Even positive life changes such as a job promotion, a new baby, or a wedding can become sources of stress in the form of added responsibility and pressure. And it doesn't have to be major sources of stress: think about how you react when you're stuck in traffic or worried about making that American Express payment for the month. Unfortunately, whether good or bad, stress shows up the same unwanted way—on your face.

Not only is stress a fact of life but also its effects are cumulative. You may have successfully handled a large, stressful event only to be bombarded by many small stressors, which add up and eventually take their toll. As we've witnessed all too often, stress can make the skin on your face drop—seemingly overnight.

At times it may seem almost impossible, but our advice is to take control of the stress in your life and relax. Here are some methods that work for us:

- *Find time each day for breathing exercises. Inhale to a slow count of ten and then exhale to an equally slow count of ten. Practice this daily and then, when a stressful situation arises, breathe.*

- *Meditate or practice self-hypnosis.*

- *Exercise, go for a walk, or practice yoga.*

- *Soak in a hot tub—but not too hot.*

- *Get a massage.*

- *Take a vacation.*

- *Get a full night's sleep.*

- *If your levels of stress seem overwhelming, seek help through a therapist.*

5. EAT RIGHT

Contrary to popular belief, eating chocolate and French fries won't give you acne, but eating a well-balanced, healthy diet will help your skin look its best. Recent research suggests that certain foods such as fresh fruits and vegetables, meats, and fish slow the aging process. Others, in particular refined carbohydrates such as flour, sugar, and milk, accelerate it.

What Supplements Do You Need?

First and foremost, it's always better to get your nutrition through your food, but if you don't eat as well as you should, take a multivitamin every day. For best absorption, take half in the morning and half at night. Make sure it includes the following:

Folic Acid (400 mcg)

Magnesium (400 mg)

Iron (10–15 mg) (unless you are postmenopausal)

omega-3 and omega-6 fatty acids

Vitamin D3 (1000 IU)

Calcium citrate (1000–1500 mg)

Since your skin is a reflection of what is going on inside your body, we recommend that you eat a balanced, healthy diet. Start by critically assessing your nutritional habits and make healthier adjustments. Stay away from processed and fast foods and, whenever possible, choose fresh, organic products. In essence, any diet deemed good for your overall health is going to be good for your skin.

- *Get enough essential fatty acids—omega-3 and omega-6—which are responsible for boosting the skin's barrier and keeping moisture in and irritants out. Good sources include salmon, sardines, walnuts, and flax seed (which needs to be finely ground in order to be properly digested).*

- *Incorporate foods rich in vitamin A (such as dark green and dark orange vegetables) and vitamin E (such as almonds and sunflower oil) into your diet for their antioxidant benefits.*

- *Eat lots of the "super" antioxidant foods such as blueberries, blackberries, and prunes to help protect your skin from free radicals.*

- *Stay away from a high glycemic diet, or foods filled with processed sugars and white flour, because in addition to not being good for your overall health, recent research shows a link between high glycemic diets and acne (see details in Chapter Eight).*

So what about dieting and the skin? We have patients who have tried the grapefruit diet, the cabbage soup diet, and the carb lover's diet; they've also experimented with South Beach, Atkins, and SlimFast and toyed with Jenny Craig, NutriSystem, and the Zone—only to lose and gain the same fifteen to twenty stubborn pounds at least a dozen times. And that yo-yo dieting shows on their skin as well.

If you're constantly losing and gaining weight, you are putting undue stress on your skin's ability to expand and contract, eventually resulting in loss of elasticity. Over and over again we observe that maintaining a fairly constant weight is just as important for your skin as the food you put into your body.

For the sake of your skin and your body, stay away from fad diets. We often refer patients to Weight Watchers because it teaches portion control, not starvation. Starvation only makes the body hold onto fat more, and certain parts of the body such as "saddlebags" are particularly diet-resistant. Portion control is a practical lifestyle choice that will serve you well in the long run. If you need to lose a significant amount of weight, consult a physician who can put you on a program that is both safe and effective. Your skin will thank you for it.

"If you eat only one vitamin-enriched fruit, make it papaya! Pound for pound, papayas contain more vitamin A than apricots, more vitamin C than oranges, and more potassium than a banana—and they taste great, too."

DR. KATHY FIELDS

⊕ Gastric Bypass and Skin

Patients who have undergone gastric bypass surgery can have special challenges associated with their skin. Without the right nutritional supplementation, skin may become pale, sallow, even gray. Additionally, the rapid weight loss associated with gastric bypass can leave skin stretched out, looking like a deflated balloon, often requiring plastic surgery to remove the redundant skin. Of course the benefits of the surgery often outweigh the health risks associated with the procedure, but it's important to be prepared for the dietary adjustments and surgery required to achieve both the health- and appearance-related benefits.

6. EXERCISE REGULARLY

Regular exercise should be an important part of every antiaging skincare program because it increases circulation, which ensures that vital nutrients are delivered to skin cells. We recommend a minimum of sixty minutes a day, four days a week, but preferably seven days a week. Consistent exercise has also been shown to reduce stress, and this, of course, is beneficial to skin. So find a cross-training exercise program you'll stick with. Ideally, incorporate both weight training and aerobic activities such as biking and swimming.

If jogging is your thing, you may want to consider switching to a lower-impact option such as biking, swimming, yoga, Pilates, weight training, or walking. Have you ever noticed that longtime runners often have a gaunt, wasted look? That's because they have very little body fat, which makes their faces look older. Additionally, regular jarring exercise may loosen and tear the microscopic attachments that bind muscle to skin, leading to sagging. Finally, if your skin has a tendency to flush during aerobic exercise, keep a cold, wet towel handy and apply it to your face during and upon completion of your exercise.

With age, stretching and including exercise forms such as yoga and Pilates into your routine become even more important to preserve balance and avoid injury. With this type of cross-training program, you'll see results in a firmer, healthier body, a glowing, younger-looking face, and a more relaxed attitude.

7. DRINK ALCOHOL ONLY IN MODERATION

While one glass of cabernet with dinner is probably harmless, in larger quantities, alcohol can damage your skin's appearance. Alcohol causes small blood vessels to dilate and increases blood flow near the surface of the skin, resulting in facial redness. Over time, the vessels can become permanently damaged, resulting in "broken capillaries" and a permanent flushed appearance of the nose and cheeks. And alcohol can trigger flare-ups of rosacea.

Alcohol also dehydrates your skin, disrupts your sleep cycle, and destroys your body's supply of vitamin A, weakening the skin's ability to fight off damage caused by free radicals. It impairs the absorption of other essential nutrients because it damages the lining of the stomach and small intestine. Just look in the mirror the morning after you've had a few too many drinks—your skin looks sallow, puffy, and dried out.

To keep your skin looking fresh, limit your alcohol consumption to no more than one drink a day. When you do have a drink, you may want to choose a glass of red wine. Researchers have found that moderate red wine consumption may be beneficial to more than just your heart. One study found that resveratrol, a polyphenol prevalent in the skin of red grapes, has powerful antioxidant benefits and may inhibit tumor development in some cancers and be helpful in the treatment of diseases such as Alzheimer's and Parkinson's. The downside of red wine, however, is a greater tendency of facial flushing.

Dermatology 911

Dermatologists are frequently called to the set of a movie. Why? Because anyone can be hit with a pimple when it is least welcome. To keep their skin looking perfect, actors and actresses receive a quick cortisone shot. It clears up a pimple in fewer than twenty-four hours. So although you may not be a celebrity, you'll want to look like one on occasions such as your wedding. If a pimple starts to surface a day or two before the big event, visit your dermatologist to quickly and easily treat your emergency.

8. FIND THE RIGHT SKINCARE ROUTINE AND STICK WITH IT

Everyone has different skincare concerns and needs, which vary depending upon the climate, your lifestyle, and your age. It's important to understand what factors influence your skin before deciding on a specific course of action.

Do for yourself what we have our patients do during their first consultation in our practices: remove all your makeup and take a good look at your skin in a 3x mirror. (Please stay away from 8x mirrors; they magnify every little line and mark that no one ever really sees.)

Take a look at your answers from the workbook section in Chapter One where you identified and prioritized your main problem areas—acne, hyperpigmentation, or aging. Remember to keep it real and not to obsess over every enlarged pore, small scar, or brown mole. Once you've completed the exercise, develop a skincare regimen that will best treat that issue. Choose products that contain specific active ingredients that address your concern and feel good to use. We learned early in our careers that compliance with a skincare program is key to achieving results. In the chapters that follow, we'll help you find the best answer for your skin.

9. DON'T BE PICKY

When a great big juicy pimple is staring back at you in the mirror, it's human nature to take action and attack. While we understand the perverse pleasure in picking and squeezing, don't do it! Popping pimples forces the bacteria deeper into the skin, causing greater inflammation. It can also lead to infections such as staph, temporary discoloration of the area, delay in healing, and, worse yet, it can leave you with scars. It's best to treat your skin with some TLC and use the right products to heal the blemish, such as topical sulfur or benzoyl peroxide. And if you can, see your dermatologist for an emergency injection. The results can be nothing short of miraculous and can truly save the day.

Habitual face picking can be part of an obsessive-compulsive personality, which is very prevalent in teenage girls and high-functioning women. If you think this might describe you, see a doctor who may suggest hypnosis, behavioral modification therapy, or antidepressant medications.

10. ADAPT YOUR SKINCARE ROUTINE TO YOUR CLIMATE

Have you ever visited the arid deserts of Palm Springs or Nevada and found everything on your body drying up? From

"Having family in both Chicago and Florida, I travel back and forth between these vastly different climates all the time. When I'm in Chicago during the winter, my hair is flat, my nails are brittle, and my skin is dry and dull, but when I go to the humidity of Florida, my hair is full and bouncy, my nails are gorgeous, and my skin is juicy. This clearly shows you what climate can do."

DR. KATHY FIELDS

your hair to your skin to your nasal membranes, you can see and feel an immediate difference when you go from a humid to an arid climate.

Or, conversely, have you ever taken a trip to a humid locale such as Miami in the summer and found your skin moist, dewy-looking, and luminous or perhaps just a bit too shiny with hair gone wild?

Maybe the skincare products you use every day feel different on your skin, too. The climate—temperature, wind, humidity, and even altitude—affects your skin, nails, and hair and impacts the efficacy of your skincare products.

Since skin is hydrated primarily from the outside rather than the inside, climate plays an important role. In regions of low humidity, the skin is dehydrated, dull, and flaky. Dry, windy climates suck moisture from the epidermis, magnifying the appearance of lines and wrinkles. High-altitude cities such as Denver filter less uv radiation, generating more free radicals to prematurely age skin. Cold weather chaps the skin, while hot weather creates a microclimate where acne thrives because of increased oil production.

We're not suggesting that you move to ensure perfect skin but rather that you evaluate your environment and adapt your skincare routine accordingly. If you're going skiing, make sure you

Tips and Tricks for Different Locales

S.O.S. for Dry, Dehydrated Skin

Avoid long, hot showers; they actually draw moisture out of your skin and make you itchy. Instead, go for tepid, quick showers. Apply a heavy moisturizer regularly after bathing or showering while skin is still damp to seal in extra moisture.

If you soak in a warm bath, we recommend using bath oil.

Use a loofah sponge or a body microdermabrasion product regularly with warm water to boost circulation and remove dead skin cells.

Use products containing humectants such as sodium hyalurante, glycolic acid, and glycerin to attract water to skin and hold onto moisture.

Keep humidity in your home at about 50% or use a humidifier.

High-Altitude Tips

Slather on extra moisturizer in the morning and at night.

uv radiation increases 10%–12% for every 3,000 feet of elevation, so even if you can't see the sun, apply sunscreen with antioxidants to protect your skin.

Don't forget to protect your lips as well. The sun can be relentless at higher altitudes, especially in states such as Colorado, where the sun shines more than three hundred days a year.

Use saline nasal sprays to keep the membranes of your nose moist and prevent nosebleeds.

Keep Your Skin Looking Fresh in the Tropics

Use a clay-based cleansing mask weekly to unclog pores and help prevent blemishes.

Heat and humidity increase oil production. Apply oil-free moisturizer only to areas of the face that feel dry and tight.

Your sunscreen comes off with your sweat, so reapply it often. Mineral sunscreens containing zinc oxide can have a mattifying effect and may work better for oily skin.

Carry oil-blotting papers to refresh your face throughout the day.

Avoid strong hydroxy acids or other ingredients that are more likely to sting skin in hot, humid environments.

wear extra sunblock to protect your skin at higher altitudes. If you live in a dry climate, apply extra moisture to your skin, especially at night when skin is receptive. If you're in a hot, humid locale, a heavy moisturizer used on acne-prone skin might make you break out.

Leading Skincare Myths

The following skincare myths are just that—myths. Educating yourself will help you better care for your skin.

MYTH: I need to drink at least eight glasses of water a day for my skin.
FACT: The outside humidity, not how much water you consume, determines how dry you are. Contrary to a popular myth perpetuated by bottled water companies, downing excessive fluids is not the best way to keep skin from drying out. In fact, by overhydrating, you will flush essential vitamins and electrolytes out of your bloodstream. You need only ninety-one ounces of fluids a day, which you can easily obtain from both food and beverages. Trust your body's natural signal: thirst. Only severe dehydration will cause your skin to dry out.

MYTH: Ninety percent of sun damage is done before you're eighteen, so it doesn't matter what I do to my skin as an adult.
FACT: Although one blistering burn when you are young can double your chances of developing skin cancer as an adult, sun damage is cumulative throughout your life. By age eighteen, you've acquired only 23% of your lifetime dose of UVA. Therefore, most of the damage has not been done. So, no excuses. Always protect yourself from harmful UV radiation.

MYTH: I have oily skin, so I'll age well.
FACT: Many factors determine how your skin ages, and skin type doesn't really play a role. Women with dry skin can achieve the same level of hydration as those with oily skin through application of moisturizers. And oily skin actually has some negatives as it ages. Oil glands may enlarge, resulting in big pores and pink/yellow growths called sebaceous hyperplasia.

MYTH: Facial exercises will lift my skin.
FACT: You can't really fight gravity. The more you make the same facial movements, the deeper your lines become. Every time the forty-four muscles in your face contract and relax, they create all sorts of facial movements. Since these muscles are attached to the skin, every time they move—when you speak, eat, laugh, or cry—your skin moves, too. Therefore, exercising your facial muscles will most likely accentuate your wrinkles.

Cut this out and put it on your bathroom mirror as a daily reminder.

Top Ten Healthy Skin Habits

1. Protect your skin from the sun
2. Don't smoke—ever!
3. Get your beauty sleep—on your back
4. Don't stress out
5. Eat right
6. Exercise regularly
7. Drink alcohol only in moderation
8. Find the right skincare routine and stick with it
9. Don't be "picky"
10. Adapt your skincare routine to your climate

MYTH: If I don't use a moisturizer, I'll get wrinkles.
FACT: The purpose of moisturizers is to hydrate dry skin and deliver a temporary smoothing benefit. Moisturizers alone do not prevent wrinkles. The best anti-wrinkle ingredients are sunscreen, retinol, glycolic acid, peptides, and acetyl glucosamine.

MYTH: Steam baths are great for skin.
FACT: They may feel refreshing and relaxing and give you a moment to de-stress, but they don't help your skin. In fact, for people with fair skin, steam baths and saunas can cause capillaries in your face to blossom, as can any activity in which you raise your body temperature. That even includes drinking hot tea or coffee.

MYTH: If washing my face once a day is good, then washing my face four times a day is great.
FACT: Overwashing disrupts the skin's delicate moisture barrier, leading to dryness, irritation, and potential flare-ups of conditions such as eczema. Skin can produce more oil following cleansing, creating a vicious cycle of oil production. In addition to a harsh cleanser stripping skin of the lipid barrier that keeps it balanced, water itself is actually very drying because it draws moisture out of the skin. We recommend using a cleanser that is right for your skin once or twice a day and then rinsing with warm water to avoid stripping skin of its natural moisturizing factors.

MYTH: I'm protected from sun damage because I wear sunscreen when I go outside.
FACT: Many people don't know that their skin can be under attack from UV rays even when sitting indoors next to a window or when driving a car. That is why wearing the right sunscreen every single day, from sunup to sundown, is so important. And don't forget to reapply.

MYTH: Aging skin is inevitable, and skin damage is irreversible without surgery.
FACT: Of course everyone ages, but the way in which your skin ages is very much under your control. A combination of healthy lifestyle habits, appropriate skincare products, and dermatologic procedures can give amazing results. For instance, the use of a hydroquinone skincare program can reverse dark marks from the sun, restoring skin's evenness and radiance.

MYTH: Your skin "gets used to" skincare products, which makes them stop working.
FACT: For most skincare products, you'll see the full extent of corrective benefits within approximately twelve weeks. The preventive benefits, on the other hand, are ongoing and difficult to measure but may be even more important for your skin than the corrective benefits. Just because you're no longer seeing the type of rapid progress you observed when you first started a regimen doesn't mean it's not working. But instead of providing the initial change you saw in your skin, it may be maintaining it at a more healthy level.

Do You Have Healthy Habits?

How many lifestyle changes do you need to make for your skin?
We've designed our own questionnaire to help you evaluate your habits
and focus on making changes for the health of your skin.

Answer "Yes" or "No" to the following:

_____ 1. Do you wear sunscreen every day outside?

_____ 2. Do you wear sunscreen when you drive or sit near a window?

_____ 3. Do you exercise at least four days a week?

_____ 4. Do you get at least eight hours of uninterrupted sleep a night?

_____ 5. Do you sleep on your back (or with a support pillow)?

_____ 6. Do you take thirty minutes each day for yourself (to meditate, do yoga, read)?

_____ 7. Do you get two to three helpings of foods rich in omega-3s or omega-6s
each week?

_____ 8. Do you eat three to five servings of leafy green and orange fruits and
vegetables a day?

_____ 9. Do you smoke cigarettes?

_____ 10. Do you drink more than one alcoholic beverage a day?

_____ 11. Do you run or jog?

_____ 12. Does your weight fluctuate more than twenty pounds?

_____ 13. Do you pick at your skin?

Scoring:

Question 1:   Yes = 5 points/No = -10 points
Questions 2-8:   Yes = 1 point/No = -2 points
Question 9:   Yes = -5 points/No = 3 points
Questions 10-12:   Yes = -2 points/No = 1 point
Question 13:   Yes = -4 points/No = 2 points

Your Healthy Habits Score:

18–20 points: Congratulations! You take great care of
yourself and it probably shows.

12–17 points: While you are taking good care of yourself,
you slip up occasionally by forgetting to use sunscreen
or indulging in unhealthy foods. Try to incorporate two
positive changes in your lifestyle over the next month.

5–11 points: You're living on the edge, setting yourself up to
look older than your years. It's time to make a commitment
to a healthier lifestyle routine. Otherwise, your options for
looking great and feeling great will diminish as damage
accumulates.

< 5 points: Whatever your age, it's never too late to start
incorporating good habits. Your future face is in your
hands, so make positive changes soon so your skin won't
have to pay the price.

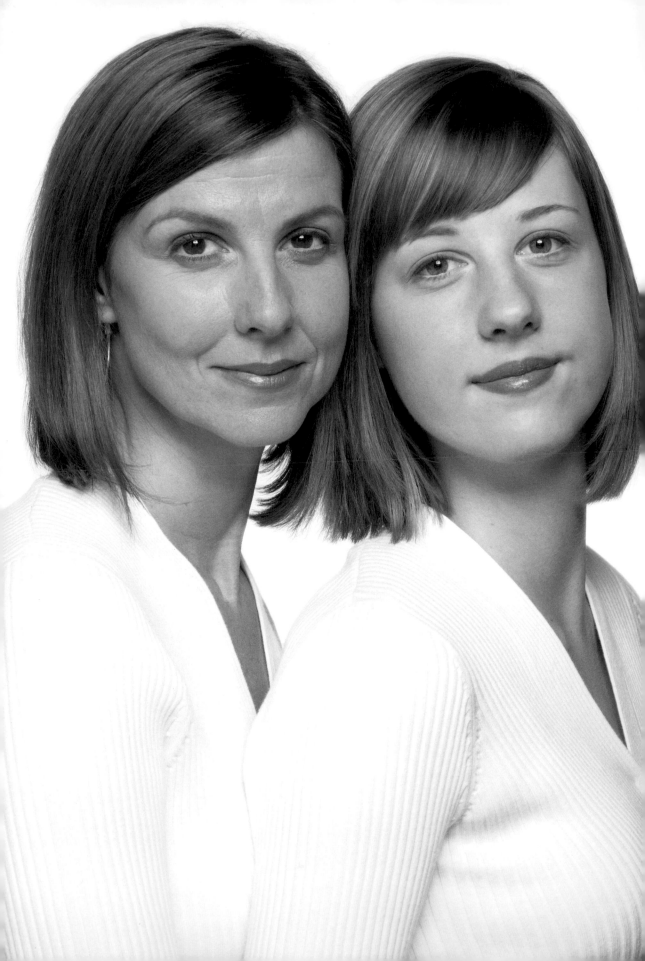

HURRICANE OF HORMONES

They Impact Your Skin at Every Age

"A period is just the beginning of a lifelong sentence."

Author Cathy Crimmins

Doctor Louann Brizendine, author of *The Female Brain*, reports that hormones are responsible for the vast majority of behavioral, emotional, and physical differences between the sexes, and this includes differences in skin, particularly as they relate to the way skin changes and ages throughout life.[1]

In this chapter, we'll outline the effects hormones have on skin throughout a woman's life and show you how to help your skin weather a lifetime of hormonal storms.

One of the marvels of human physiology is the extent to which our gender identity is tied to substances secreted by our glands and tissues called hormones. Men and women are uniquely different creatures because of hormonal differences that shape us from our first fetal weeks in the womb through adolescence and into our golden years.

Scientists have discovered that the impact of sex-related hormones starts at approximately eight weeks after conception. Males experience a surge in testosterone while females are drenched in hormones such as estrogen, progesterone, and oxytocin and neurotransmitters such as dopamine and serotonin. So at a mere eight weeks of gestation, we go our separate ways gender-wise, and there's no turning back.

Hormones have power over every cell in our bodies, and nowhere is that power more visible than in the skin. In early childhood, the differences in the skin of girls and boys may not be obvious. However, with the onset of puberty, sex hormones skyrocket, ruling behavior and altering the appearance of skin, hair, and nails. After surviving this pubertal hormonal assault, men's hormones continue in a steady state from hour to hour and day to day.

On the other hand, female hormones fluctuate dramatically throughout the month, exerting control over all aspects of a woman's life. Thanks to their unrelenting influence, we can wake up elated one morning and irritated the next. We may be humming along at work, feeling good, and then, whammo, be blindsided by a headache.

And we cannot ignore the interplay between hormone-related emotions and our sense of self-confidence. Our appearance can truly be affected by our mood. We all know it's difficult to project beauty and strength when a bombardment of hormones leaves us with an inexplicable feeling of impending doom.

The Major Hormones That Impact Our Skin, Hair, and Nails

ESTROGEN	MELANIN
Used throughout the female body, estrogen maintains the health of the brain, blood vessels, reproductive organs, urinary tract, breasts, bones, and skin.	Stimulating hormone: secreted by the pituitary gland, this hormone regulates skin pigmentation.

PROGESTERONE	CORTISOL
Serves many vital functions, such as maintaining pregnancy and regulating menstrual cycles. It also has diuretic properties and enhances the beneficial effects of estrogen while preventing problems linked to estrogen excess such as uterine cancer. In some people, progesterone may cause moodiness.	Produced by the adrenal glands, cortisol controls the stress response and glucose metabolism and impacts immune function. If you live a highly stressful life, the effects of cortisol can be very destructive, leading to severe strain on virtually all your organs.

THYROID HORMONES	TESTOSTERONE
The family of hormones secreted by the thyroid gland affects the metabolism of every cell in your body. Imbalances in these hormones lead to weight gain or loss, body temperature fluctuations, depression, hair loss or hair growth, and dry skin. As we age, our thyroid hormones decrease.	An anabolic hormone that builds and maintains bone and muscle mass, skin elasticity, sex drive, and cardiovascular health in both sexes.

The Beauty of Hormones: How They Affect Appearance

Let's take a closer look at hormonal influences on skin, hair, and nails during various stages of a woman's life.

The Teen Years

The power and presence of hormones explodes during puberty. According to ecologist and author Sandra Steingraber in *The Falling Age of Puberty*, the onset of pubescent physical changes is starting at a younger and younger age.[2] In fact, Steingraber notes that adolescent breast development is occurring in girls, on average, one to two years earlier than it did just forty years ago.

The physical transformation that occurs during puberty can, at times, be unattractive and emotionally bewildering. From acne and body odor to stretch marks, dandruff, and moles, hormones wreak havoc on teens at a time when self-esteem is fragile.

With the arrival of menstruation, teenage girls face bigger challenges from their hormones than boys. The hormonal surges that accompany menses frequently cause moodiness, bloating, cramps, and acne, which often extend beyond puberty, plaguing us until menopause.

Society has us believing that because acne and dandruff are a common occurrence associated with life's transitions, they are to be tolerated and endured. As dermatologists, we don't accept this tenet and want to alleviate some of the physical and emotional scars these conditions can cause. Below, we suggest easy, therapeutic approaches to some common troubling skin problems triggered by "teen" hormones.

> **? DID YOU KNOW?**
>
> 41% OF WOMEN EXPERIENCE PREMENSTRUAL BREAKOUTS.[3]

ACNE

WHAT IS IT? Inflamed lesions on the skin triggered by androgenic hormones including testosterone and DHEA-S, among others. The effect of hormones is to increase the secretion of sticky oil in the hair follicle. When mixed with dead skin cells, this produces a plug, the initial event in the acne cycle.

WHAT CAN YOU DO? In addition to treatments for acne described in Chapter Eight, prescription birth control pills such as Yaz are also very effective in controlling breakouts because they help to mitigate the impact of hormonal fluctuations on skin. Remember that acne isn't curable and often lasts many years. So, once you get it under control, you must stick with a daily skincare program to maintain your clear skin.

CELLULITE

WHAT IS IT? Cellulite is a deposit of fat that pushes against the connective tissue just below the surface of the skin, causing skin to look dimply and puckered like an orange peel or cottage cheese. It is not specifically related to being overweight. In fact, many thin women battle these troublesome dimples. It can appear as early as the teen years because hormones play a key role

The Younger Acne Begins, the More Severe It Becomes

Two large clinical studies of teenage boys and girls conducted by pediatric dermatologist Dr. Anne W. Lucky, the director of the dermatology clinic at the Children's Hospital Medical Center in Cincinnati, Ohio, determined that the earlier acne begins, the greater the likelihood that it will become more severe with age. As reported in the *Journal of Pediatrics* and the *Archives of Dermatology*, the studies evaluated the severity of acne over a five-year period and found that the subjects with acne lesions at the start (age nine or ten) had the most severe acne at age fifteen. Therefore, the researchers concluded that effective recognition and treatment would help prevent and lessen the severity and reduce chances of scarring in early-onset acne.[4, 5]

in its formation. While estrogen appears to initiate the development of cellulite, other hormones including insulin, cortisol, and thyroid may play a role.

WHAT CAN YOU DO? Unfortunately, there isn't a lot you can do to truly combat cellulite. However, it tends to be more common in overweight teens, so weight loss and exercise may help. Cellulite creams with xanthine, caffeine, and aminophylin may improve the appearance but must be used regularly. Thermage laser performed by a dermatologist is showing promise as a long-term treatment. There are also a few ways to camouflage cellulite, which we'll share with you later in this chapter.

DANDRUFF AND SEBORRHEIC DERMATITIS

WHAT IS IT? Like acne, seborrheic dermatitis is initiated by androgenic hormones and is a common inflammatory disease of the skin known as dandruff in its mildest form. It appears as red, inflamed patches covered by oily or dry scales that may feel chapped or itchy. It can be found on the scalp, eyebrows, nose folds, temples, and beard area. When localized on the face, we refer to it as "facial dandruff." It can be caused by excessive oil production brought on by hormones or stress, a change in environment, or an inflammatory reaction to yeast. Dandruff is often worse in the winter because of the lack of humidity. Like many skin conditions, there is a genetic component, so if your parents suffer with it, you are more prone to experience it as well.

WHAT CAN YOU DO? There are very effective over-the-counter medicated shampoos and creams to treat seborrheic dermatitis and dandruff. The active ingredients approved for dandruff treatment by the United States Food and Drug Administration (FDA) include tar, pyrithione zinc, salicylic acid, selenium sulfide, sulfur, and ketoconazole. Cortisone creams are also beneficial for reducing inflammation and can be purchased over the counter in doses up to 1%. For extreme cases, you may want to see your dermatologist for a prescription-strength shampoo or cream.

MOLES

WHAT IS IT? Medically known as melanocytic nevi, moles are small dark spots on your skin that, according to the American Academy of Dermatology, appear predominately during the first twenty years of life. Only one in one hundred babies is born with them, while most adults have an average of twenty moles. Hormones, sun exposure, and genetics are all factors in the number, location, and type of moles we each get. In particular, hormonal surges during puberty cause new moles to appear and existing moles to darken.

WHAT CAN YOU DO? UV light exposure can trigger the onset of moles, darken their appearance, and possibly cause a malignant transformation, so protect them with sunscreen or clothing. Many moles can be surgically removed quite easily, which is something to consider if you are bothered by their cosmetic appearance. Additionally, you should have your moles checked by a doctor regularly to rule out melanoma, especially if you notice a change in color, size, or shape or if a new mole appears. We will discuss moles in more depth in Chapter Eleven.

SWEATING AND BODY ODOR

WHAT IS IT? Anyone who lives with a teenage boy is quite familiar with sweat and body odor. Once we hit puberty, boys and girls alike start to perspire from exercise, heat, and anxiety. Sweating is natural, but the quantity and particular odor vary widely and can be attributed to medical conditions, some foods and beverages, mood, hormone levels, and bacterial overgrowth on the surface of the skin. Perspiration triggered by hormones often causes people to sweat on their faces, armpits, palms, feet, and torsos. Excessive sweating, a condition known as hyperhidrosis, creates an environment that is ripe for the growth of bacteria, fungus, and yeast, often contributing to conditions

Deodorants versus Antiperspirants: What's the Difference?

Although many people use the terms interchangeably, deodorants and antiperspirants work quite differently. Deodorants do not stop perspiration. Instead, they contain antiseptic ingredients that target the bacteria in sweat, which causes the odor. They also contain fragrance to mask the odor that does occur. The result: the smell associated with sweating is neutralized. Antiperspirants, on the other hand, partially stop the body from producing sweat by clogging the sweat glands. The result: you don't perspire as much. Some antiperspirants may also contain antibacterial agents in the formula. Deodorants and antiperspirants work best when applied to dry skin.

such as dandruff and foot fungus. There are a few who don't need an antiperspirant at all, but for the majority …

WHAT CAN YOU DO? For those who perspire heavily, start by applying an over-the-counter antiperspirant daily, both in the morning and at night on dry, clean skin. If you are experiencing hyperhidrosis, check with your doctor, who may prescribe a stronger antiperspirant such as Drysol Dab-O-Matic. Antiperspirants create a plug in the sweat gland that blocks sweat from being released. They are completely safe and have been used effectively for decades. For the best results, and to avoid irritation, apply an antiperspirant to dry skin. In some cases, your doctor may even suggest Botox injections for affected areas, which work well to stop perspiration, helping to eliminate bacteria and yeast. We also encourage teens to experiment with different deodorants to mask unpleasant odors.

TELANGIECTASIAS

WHAT IS IT? Often referred to as "broken capillaries," they aren't really broken. Rather, telangiectasias are small, dilated new vessels under the skin's surface that are offshoots from deeper blood vessels. Telangiectasias can be triggered by hormones, topical agents such as Retin-A, activities such as hot saunas, or sunbathing. They may appear in children as young as eight to ten, are fairly common in teens, and are far more visible in fair-skinned individuals. You can expect the telangiectasias that present during puberty to disappear spontaneously after a few years. Unfortunately, adult-onset telangiectasias do not disappear on their own.

WHAT CAN YOU DO? Attracted to the red color in the vessel, green lasers weld the visible vein shut. However, laser treatment may not be a permanent solution because it will not stop new vessels from forming. Retreatment after a year or so is often necessary. While we have not found topical agents such as vitamin K effective, avoidance of exacerbating practices such as steam baths, saunas, and overly aggressive exfoliation may lessen the likelihood of reemergence.

> **DID YOU KNOW?**
>
> ANY TIME YOUR FACE GETS BEET RED, WHETHER FROM EXERCISE, STEAM BATHS, OR DRINKING HOT BEVERAGES, YOU ARE AT RISK OF DILATING BLOOD VESSELS. SUCK ON ICE CHIPS OR KEEP A COOL TOWEL HANDY DURING EXERCISE.

The Midyears, or Perimenopause: When Hormones Start to Let Us Down

The way we think about middle age has shifted dramatically. Our life expectancy in 1900 was forty-seven. Now that's just the halfway mark. Therefore, today we need to deal with the hormonal complications of menopause when we're feeling far from old.

The physical changes that occur during our late forties through our fifties can be very disconcerting, to say the least. Men are biologically hardwired to notice women when we are at the peak of fertility. They are attracted to us when our skin is flawless, our cheeks are soft and round, and our lips are shaped like rosebuds. They admire us when our eyebrows are arched and we have a dainty waist-to-hip ratio. Once our prime fertile years are behind us, the reduction in female hormones causes significant changes in appearance—fat redistributes from our face to our fanny, our eyebrows flatten, and our lips lose their red color and plump volume. Dwindling hormone levels, coupled with cumulative sun damage, further cause our skin to get blotchy and thinner. What's more, our skeleton starts to shrink and our hair turns gray. We literally start to vanish.

Since people are no longer calling it quits at sixty-five, we need to stay in the game throughout our lives. Many of us aspire to continue our careers into our seventies and beyond, while some may find themselves in new relationships or marriages quite late in life. To help us lead the best possible lives, it's important to look our best until our final days.

As dermatologists, we want to help you go the distance in peak performance and enjoy great skin at every age. Skin can be beautiful when it is nurtured, well cared for, and sun protected. Looking good until your one-hundredth birthday is something that is achievable and will make life's exciting ride ever so much more wonderful.

THE BARE BONES ON OSTEOPOROSIS

The skeleton is the framework for everything that sits on top of it. If your bones shrink, your eye sockets hollow and your skin hangs. Therefore, it's important to take care of your skeletal foundation to keep your skin looking tight.

Osteoporosis is a disease characterized by a loss of bone mass resulting in brittle bones that easily break. Studies have shown that bone mass begins to diminish after the age of thirty-five to forty as a result of the decline in estrogen hormones. The rate of loss dramatically accelerates in the years following menopause.

How common is osteoporosis? In October of 2004, the u.s. Surgeon General warned that ten million Americans over the age of fifty have osteoporosis, while another thirty-four million are at risk for developing the bone disease, with women four times more likely to develop the disease than men.[6]

We actually think that osteoporosis is underdiagnosed, particularly in men. National research has found that bone mass declines for all of us during our adult years, which is why it is so important to adopt preventive measures.

Because osteoporosis is asymptomatic, most people don't have their first bone density test until after forty, at which time they are often shocked to learn how much loss they have already experienced. Don't wait for your doctor to order a bone density test. Schedule one proactively, particularly if osteoporosis runs in your family or you have a history of anorexia.

And don't forget that just like your bones, your teeth also provide structure for your lips and face. If they aren't healthy, your face won't look its best.

Taking calcium and magnesium daily and doing weight-bearing exercises can prevent osteoporosis. It's ideal to begin both as early in life as possible, but no matter what your age, you should incorporate them into your daily routine. Your doctor can also offer additional remedies that maintain bone density and build strong, healthy bones.

Why Anorexia Nervosa Makes Young People Look Old

A poor diet contributes to the onset of osteoporosis. According to an article in the *Journal of the American Medical Association*, 50% of young patients with the eating disorder anorexia nervosa were diagnosed with premature osteoporosis.[7] Studies have shown that 40% of skeletal calcium should be established during teenage years and peak bone mass (PBM) is reached at around the age of twenty. Unfortunately, that is the most common age for females to be afflicted with eating disorders.

Along with the impact on skeletal health, starvation associated with anorexia nervosa also has a profound effect on skin, with loss of underlying fat tissue causing sagging and lack of nutrients causing pallor, extreme frailness, and increased body hair growth.

I NEVER HAD ACNE AS A TEENAGER—WHY NOW?

During their reproductive years, women have a natural balance between the masculinizing androgenic hormones such as progesterone and the feminizing hormone estrogen. Beginning in our thirties, a natural reduction in estrogen causes the ratio of estrogens to androgens to decrease. In other words, our feminine hormones begin disappearing, and our masculine ones may be increasing. So the scale tips in favor of the masculinizing androgens. As a result, our sebaceous glands secrete thicker sebum, which clogs the pores and produces acne in some adult women. This acne is not short-lived. In fact, medical studies have documented that adult female acne lasts, on average, twenty years.

> "What a shock it was to learn that my strong, healthy husband has borderline osteoporosis. The same way that women are often overlooked for risk of heart disease, men are overlooked when it comes to osteoporosis. Our advice to men is to have their bone density checked as well."
>
> **DR. KATIE RODAN**

This acne may affect the body as well as the face. The countless hours spent running on the treadmill, lifting weights, and posing in downward-facing dog to get your body in its best shape may actually be causing the pimple that just appeared on your back. Heat, friction, sweat, and tight clothing, many of the elements involved in working out, are just what acne needs to thrive and flourish. And although body acne is not usually cocktail party conversation, it is surprisingly prevalent. It's important to us that every inch of a woman's skin looks great so she can walk with confidence, whether wearing an evening dress or a bathing suit.

If you are prone to body acne, we recommend cleansing immediately after exercising with a medicated body wash and applying a salicylic acid treatment (it won't bleach clothes or bedding) to help keep skin fresh and clear.

Additionally, middle age is a time when many women consider discontinuing birth control pills. Realize that if you do, acne may rear its ugly head. Since acne can be a problem in the perimenopausal years, we recommend talking to your internist or gynecologist about starting or continuing oral contraceptives. This can help regulate fluctuating hormones to maintain your sanity and a clearer complexion as well.

THE YIN AND YANG OF ESTROGEN

Estrogen, which defines our beautiful, feminine characteristics, is also responsible for some of the physical challenges that women seem to experience more than men. Estrogen stimulates localized fat deposits especially around the abdomen, thighs, back, and buttocks. And unfortunately, we gain fat in our waistline, increasing our risk of heart disease. On the thighs, fat doesn't just settle; it presses through collagen fibers in the skin, helping cellulite to blossom even on the skinniest bodies. Unlike men, 90% of women will have some cellulite by age seventy.

How can you ward off the curse of cottage cheese thighs? To start with, cellulite is less noticeable on darker skin, so self-tanners may reduce the appearance of the dimples. Additionally, cellulite creams containing caffeine and xanthine may temporarily decrease the size of fat lobules, improving the appearance of cellulite. However, they offer no long-term solution. Some controversial treatments for cellulite include mesotherapy, injections of vitamins or other ingredients such as phosphotidylcholine into the cellulite, but these treatments are unproven and may carry risks including pain, swelling, redness, and draining cysts. Liposuction is not effective either since it targets fat deep below the skin's surface, bypassing the more superficial cellulite layer.

Although there is no cure at present, we are excited about the ongoing research in this area with promising developments in laser and ultrasonic technology that may prove fruitful in the years to come. Until then, work on fighting a growing midriff and controlling that redistribution of fat that occurs during your midlife years. Sign up for an abs class, take up belly dancing, or try thirty minutes of Hoola-hoop a day. Exercise keeps your muscles toned, helps shed unwanted pounds, reduces stress, and is great for bone density, so incorporate it into your life.

Menopause, the Hormonal Sunset

Menopause is the medical term defined as the first year after a woman's last menstrual cycle. While men experience a slow decline in testosterone, for women the decline in estrogen is very abrupt. The average age of menopause is fifty-one, but it may occur anytime from the thirties to the early sixties. Perimenopause is the precursor to menopause, typically lasting four to six years, and postmenopause refers to the years following menopause. This process may start gradually with occasional night sweats, irritability, mood swings, insomnia, and loss of libido, progressing like a freight train over the next several years as estrogen rapidly declines.

As dermatologists, we see the physical manifestations of perimenopause and menopause such as dry skin, wrinkling, acne, thinning hair, brittle nails, and overall weight gain. Here are some of the other most common complaints we hear from our patients:

DEPRESSION

Hormonally related depression is a common problem affecting approximately 25% of adult women. Women who suffer from depression during menopause often have experienced hormonal-related depression earlier in life, whether postpartum or related to their menstrual cycles. It's rare that depression surfaces for the first time during menopause; however, mood swings in perimenopause are quite common because of the hormonal fluctuations. In our practices, we've seen time and again that how you feel affects the way you look and vice versa. It's a vicious cycle but one that you can break with the proper treatment.

Remember that no matter what you may hear, you can't "think your way" out of depression. Depression is a serious condition that can be treated with medications or therapy. Therefore, recognizing the symptoms and following up with appropriate treatment is key for your future well-being. (See box on the next page for symptoms.)

Symptoms of Depression in Women[8]

- Persistent sad, anxious, or "empty" mood
- Loss of interest or pleasure in activities, including sex
- Restlessness, irritability, or excessive crying
- Feelings of guilt, worthlessness, helplessness, hopelessness, or pessimism
- Sleeping too much or too little, early-morning awakening
- Appetite and/or weight loss or overeating and weight gain
- Decreased energy, fatigue, feeling "slowed down"
- Thoughts of death or suicide or suicide attempts
- Difficulty concentrating, remembering, or making decisions
- Persistent physical symptoms that do not respond to treatment such as headaches, digestive disorders, and chronic pain

DIGESTIVE ISSUES

The thyroid gland exerts significant influence over digestive health. With age, as your thyroid hormones slow down, the gastrointestinal tract follows, causing constipation, gas, and bloating. Additionally, as people age, their gut flora deteriorates and lactose intolerance may ensue. Try taking fiber supplements along with probiotics, live cultures clinically proven to restore the balance of gut flora. Together they can improve digestive health and boost your immunity.

SKIN DRYNESS AND SKIN CELL TURNOVER

Dryness and menopause go hand in hand. With the decline in hormone production, secretions from tear ducts and the salivary and sebaceous glands slow. The end result is dryness of the eyes, mouth, vagina, and skin. Further compounding the problem, skin cell reproduction slows, causing an overall thin and crepey texture. Dead cells accumulate on the surface, causing the skin to look dull, drab, and sallow. Decreased glandular secretions and diminished cell turnover compromise natural barrier function, causing irritation and itching.

Both chemical and physical exfoliation help increase epidermal cell turnover. Chemical exfoliants are ingredients such as glycolic acid, lactic acid, and salicylic acid. If you have sensitive skin, consider products with acetyl glucosamine. All of these work by dissolving the bonds between cells in the outermost layer of skin, allowing for effective shedding of dead cells. Physical exfoliants manually slough away dead or excess skin cells. These include abrasive pads, textured sponges, and cleansers containing polyethylene beads. Exfoliation can make your skin look refreshed and renewed. Exfoliation also ensures better penetration of wrinkle fighters and medicines for acne and brown spots. That's why we are loyal fans of daily gentle chemical or physical exfoliation.

FAT, COLLAGEN, AND ELASTIN REDUCTION

It is emotionally and physically deflating to experience the reduction in skin's structural components as we age. In our forties and fifties, skin starts to wrinkle, droop, and sag seemingly overnight. Lack of hormones and cumulative sun damage result in a net loss of collagen and elastin fibers. In other words, fewer of these supporting tissues are being made to replace what is being broken down.

For example, an astounding 30% of skin collagen is lost in the first five years after menopause. Additionally, like a deflated balloon, the redistribution of fat from the face to the fanny accounts for some of the most profound changes in the aging face.

HOT FLASHES AND FLUSHES

The hot flash, or what we like to refer to as the "power surge," can come out of the blue or be triggered by something as minor as an embarrassing joke or a slight increase in room temperature. More than two-thirds of American women experience hot flashes, which are unpredictable and vary in intensity from mildly bothersome to downright uncomfortable. They can even be embarrassing for some, as beads of sweat drip off your face. The "flush blush" reddening of the face, neck, and upper chest lasts for thirty seconds to five minutes and is due to capillary dilation.

Although the exact reason for hot flashes is unknown, they are largely thought to be the result of instability of the hypothalamus, the part of the brain that regulates body temperature, plus declining estrogen. The estrogen collapse is particularly bad at night, between the hours of 2:00 a.m. and 6:00 a.m., when a woman can have hot flashes every twenty minutes. They can completely disrupt sleep, adding more stress to the body and often increasing irritability during the day, which affects your health in the long run. If you are experiencing bothersome hot flashes, seek the advice of a gynecologist sooner rather than later.

HAIR AND NAIL GROWTH AND THINNING

Many menopausal women experience hair problems, losing hair where they want it and growing it where they don't. Approximately one-third of postmenopausal women experience alopecia, hair loss at the front or top of the scalp, creating a widening of the central part. Others may experience hirsutism, or increased hair growth on the face, especially on the chin and upper lip.

Men have unusual hair growth during their older years as well. Their eyebrows, nose hairs, and ear hair becomes dark, thick, and unruly. Laser hair removal can be an extremely effective solution for unwanted dark hair in light-complexioned individuals, but beware—it doesn't work well on gray hair.

During menopause, nail growth slows, and the nail plate becomes more fragile and ridged. On the flip side, toenails become thicker, difficult to cut, and more prone to nail fungus.

? DID YOU KNOW?

SHIN GUARDS AREN'T JUST FOR SOCCER. WHEN PATIENTS SUFFER REPEATED BRUISING ON THEIR LOWER LEGS FROM BUMPING INTO COFFEE TABLES, DISHWASHERS, AND THE LIKE, WE RECOMMEND PURCHASING COTTON PADDED SHIN GUARDS TO PROTECT THEIR LEGS AT HOME AND TO MINIMIZE BRUISING AND DISCOMFORT.

BRUISING

Most people don't recognize that the dark splotches on the forearms and the back of the hands are the result of bruising from even the most minor trauma. It can start as early as the midfifties, worsening decade by decade. Eventually, this makes many people feel fragile. It is one of the many stigmas associated with aging, and our patients hate it.

It is interesting to note that this kind of bruising occurs much more frequently in areas where our skin has been constantly exposed to the sun. Sun damage weakens the collagen in the skin that anchors blood vessels, making them more prone to injury. This is one more reason why lifelong sun protection is merited. Because arms and legs are most often in motion and getting banged up, bruising results.

The good news is that bruising may be lessened and improved, though not completely eliminated. Bioflavinoids purchased at health food stores may help, but check with your physician to see whether they could interfere with other medications. Topical retinoids may thicken weak areas of skin by renewing collagen. Herbal supplements such as Arnica may be of value prior to procedures or surgery to prevent bruising and swelling. Finally, using self-tanners can mask and camouflage bruises. We like the self-tanning moisturizers that camouflage the bruising while treating dry skin.

CAN YOU TELL THEM APART?
A study of 149 female identical twins, conducted by plastic surgeon Dr. Bahman Guyuron, found that the use of hormone replacement therapy impacted the visible appearance of people with identical genes.[10]

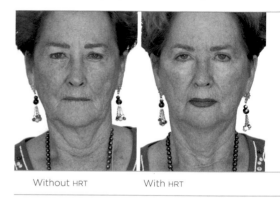

Without HRT   With HRT

Menopausal Remedies to the Rescue

We've described some pretty uncomfortable and unattractive skin, hair, and nail issues for perimenopausal and menopausal women. However, we don't want you to despair, because hormone replacement therapy (HRT) can keep you looking great. Three common prescriptions are used in HRT: estrogen therapy, progesterone replacement, and combined estrogen-progesterone therapy (EPT). It's important to speak to your gynecologist or menopause expert about which option might be suitable for you, as there are medical advantages and concerns related to each.

On the positive side, HRT reduces your risk of heart attack and osteoporosis. It keeps your brain sharp, reduces hair growth on your face, and keeps skin juicy by preserving collagen. However, HRT may not be recommended for women who are at a high risk for breast cancer or for women who are breast cancer survivors. A 2003 study in the *Journal of the American Medical Association* found that women who had been taking estrogen/progesterone were at a higher risk of developing breast cancer, even years after they stopped the treatments.[9] When you are researching symptoms and solutions, a tremendous resource is www.menopause.org, which provides the most recent options and studies available on various treatments.

What about Natural Alternatives: Bioidentical Hormone Replacement Therapy (BHRT)

Bioidentical hormone replacement therapies differ from conventional HRTs in that they are derived from plants rather than chemicals. They also differ because HRTs are manufactured by pharmaceutical companies and packaged into specific, standard doses while BHRTs are prescribed in person-specific doses and custom blended by compounding pharmacists. While producers of BHRTs claim they are "all-natural" pills and creams, this therapy is highly controversial. In fact, the FDA has recently stated that it feels BHRTs mislead women. Even so, there has been very little scientific research on the efficacy or long-term health implications of taking BHRTs. Natural healers have embraced this solution, while the medical community feels there needs to be significant research before supporting this option. Our advice is that rather than taking this into your own hands, you should proceed with caution and your doctor's advice.

But Wait—There's More

Here are some other ways to improve your looks at any age:

1. Teeth whiteners
You can lift years off your looks by whitening stains from your teeth, and it's one of the easiest things to do.

2. Combination therapies
Many procedures or medicated skin treatments can be enhanced with cosmetic or cosmeceutical treatments. For instance, pharmaceuticals such as hydroquinone have a dramatic impact on reducing brown spots, while nutritional ingredients such as soy and green tea extract exhibit anti-inflammatory and antioxidant properties. Injections such as Botox and Sculptra are very effective in eliminating deeper wrinkles and may be combined with Retin-A to help plump up collagen and add strength to skin.

3. Update your hair
If you felt like a million dollars when you left the hair salon as a twenty-year-old, you will feel great coming out at seventy, eighty, and beyond. Hair color takes years off your looks, and a flattering style can update your entire appearance. If you are worried about a sensitive scalp, ask your stylist to use foils so that the hair color doesn't come into contact with your skin.

4. Care for your hands
Hands can really give away your biological age. Our hands are often overexposed to the sun and therefore show age spots more readily than other areas of our bodies. While you are caring for your facial sunspots, don't forget to use brightening products with ingredients such as vitamin C, kojic acid and retinol on the backs of your hands.

5. Exercise
Remember, too, that controlled studies have demonstrated that exercise can reduce your biological age. Additionally, exercise releases endorphins, which elevate your mood while burning calories, helping you combat the fat redistribution that occurs during menopause.

6. Lengthen your lashes
Long, full eyelashes draw attention to the eye. As we age, our eyelashes become shorter, thinner, and more sparse. Batting thick, luscious lashes amps up your sex appeal. Need proof? Mascara is the number one selling cosmetic and has been for decades. Get the same results without the mess of mascara with Latisse®. This prescription topical medication will lengthen and thicken your lashes when used as prescribed by your dermatologist.

Don't Let the Hurricane Blow You Away

Dr. Katie Rodan's Aunt Diane is still a knockout and is one confident lady. In her own words, "At eighty-three I look better than most women at fifty-three, and I'm twice as smart as they are." Aunt Diane's healthy attitude, shared by Katie's mom, Bern, age eighty-one, comes from their lifelong commitment to caring for themselves both physically and mentally. They are both spiffy dressers with excellent posture who exercise regularly and still work! They are among the many inspirational and beautiful women we admire.

The fact is that we have many patients who maintain excellent lifestyle habits well into their nineties and still look gorgeous. We can't say this enough: be proactively involved in your health and well-being to get ahead of the game when it comes to managing the impact of hormones on your appearance.

⮞ Are Hormones the Hidden Culprit Behind Your Skin Issues?

1. Do you break out around your period?

_____ Yes   _____ No

2. In the past few months, have you started or stopped using the birth control pill?

_____ Yes   _____ No

3. Are you pregnant or have you given birth in the past three months?

_____ Yes   _____ No

4. Are you premenopausal?

_____ Yes   _____ No

5. Are you postmenopausal?

_____ Yes   _____ No

6. Are you on hormone replacement therapy (HRT)?

_____ Yes   _____ No

If you answered "Yes" to one or more of the above questions, your skin issues may be hormone related. Consult your dermatologist or ob-gyn to get to the bottom of this today.

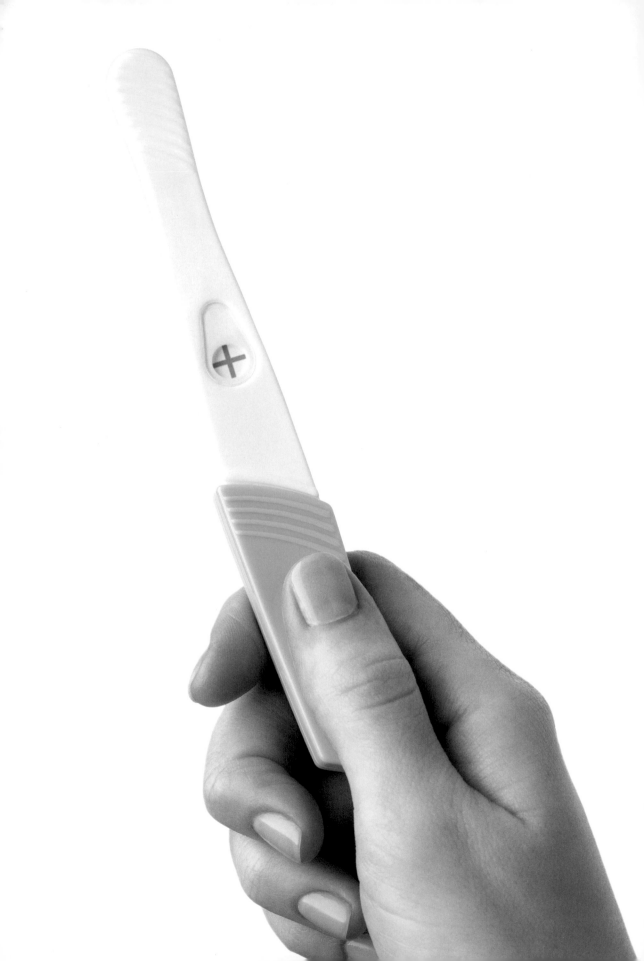

PREGNANCY
A New Definition of "Normal"

"Oh, the things you're never told about pregnancy. My son is the light of my life, but the production process was not the 'glowing' experience I had always envisioned. Moles, melasma, and other unnecessary changes popped up everywhere."

Anonymous

Nature's goal for the human female is procreation. Arguably, it's one of the most normal events in a woman's lifetime. Yet laboratory medicine explicitly tells us that when the female body converts into an incubator for a new life, our physiology changes substantially and most "normal" ranges for blood chemistry no longer apply. The same is true for our skin, where many pregnancy-related changes are visible for the whole world to see.

There Really Is a Glow—and so Much More

It's not just the joy of expecting a new baby that makes a woman's face luminous; there is actually a scientific origin to that glow. Pregnant women produce between 30%–50% more blood than nonpregnant women. The result: skin appears brighter, pinker, and more vibrant. And that's just the beginning. Because of the profound hormonal changes that occur during pregnancy, nothing is quite the same. From thicker hair and strange discolorations on your skin to protruding veins and an itchy belly, you probably notice something new almost every day. On the next few pages, we'll take a look at some of the most common dermatologic changes women experience during pregnancy and give you tips to help weather the storm.

Am I Going Bald?

Let's start with your hair, which often looks thicker and more luxurious during pregnancy. This added volume is due to a slowing of the natural shedding process rather than an increase in hair growth. For both pregnant and nonpregnant women, there are three stages in the life cycle of hair: anagen, catagen, and telogen. In nonpregnant individuals, approximately 85%–90% of hair is in the anagen, or growing, stage, while the other 5%–15% is in the catagen, or resting, stage. The remaining hair is in the telogen stage, whereby it falls out and is replaced by new growth. On average, nonpregnant women shed about one hundred hairs a day.

During pregnancy, higher levels of estrogen extend the growing stage, so fewer hairs are resting in catagen or falling out in telogen. About three months after giving birth, women experience an abrupt drop in circulating hormones, which in turn triggers a shift into the telogen stage, a condition called telogen effluvium. For some women, this loss can be massive, creating a hysterical fear of going bald. We reassure these new moms that it's just the hairs' natural growth process getting back in sync. Since we each have an average of 100,000 hairs on our heads, more than 50% loss is required before we would appear bald.

To the relief of many women, balding rarely occurs with telogen effluvium. A few weeks to months after the onset of telogen effluvium, hair shedding begins to lessen and new short hairs appear. During this normalization process, you may find your hair getting thinner than usual. If you are not breastfeeding, Rogaine (minoxidil), a topical nonprescription hair growth medicine, may help stabilize and normalize the hair cycle faster.

Speaking of hair, during pregnancy an increase in androgens (male-type hormones) may cause you to see thicker and darker hair growth on your body, which can be removed by waxing or shaving.

The Most Common Skin Issues During Pregnancy

Stretch marks (striae)	Acne
Mask of pregnancy, also referred to as melasma, the discoloration of the pigment on your face	Darkening of freckles, moles, and other areas of your skin
Varicose and spider veins on the legs	Linea nigra
Telangiectasias, or spider veins, on the face or body	Dry, itchy abdomen
	Skin tags

Pregnancy and delivery can also result in iron-deficient anemia, which may cause brittle nails, pale skin, and hair loss. Ask your doctor to check your iron levels following delivery. If your iron is low, a daily iron supplement will reverse this type of anemia.

What's Happening to My Skin?

It's not just your belly that changes during pregnancy. Every inch of your skin from your head to your toes experiences changes that are unexpected and, at times, disconcerting.

MELASMA

The "mask of pregnancy," or melasma, is the most visible manifestation of the effect of hormones on the skin during pregnancy. Melasma appears as symmetrical dark brown patches on the cheeks, upper lip, and forehead. It results from the overproduction of melanin triggered by estrogenic hormones in concert with sun exposure. Heat that comes from activities like "slaving over a hot stove" can also induce melasma, as was reported in a group of Latina kitchen workers. While it affects women of all ethnicities, darker complexions tend to have the most persistent forms.

Melasma is very disturbing for the women who see it during pregnancy, and unfortunately, it doesn't always disappear spontaneously after giving birth. Strict daily sun protection during your pregnancy is your best defense in preventing melasma. Use a broad-spectrum UVA and UVB blocker every day. If you do experience melasma, pigment-fading treatment with a medication called hydroquinone is quite effective but should be delayed until delivery and nursing are behind you.

DARKENING OF MOLES

While pregnant, you may also experience a darkening of your moles, freckles, and nipples due to changes in your skin pigmentation. A brown-pigmented streak from your belly button to your pubis, called linea nigra, is also a frequent finding starting around the fifth month of pregnancy; this may persist up to a year following delivery, and there is nothing you can do to prevent it. Even with this supercharged pigment activity, take comfort in knowing there is no increased risk of melanoma during pregnancy. However, if you notice that a specific mole or freckle is changing in color, size, or shape, you should contact your health care provider for a definitive diagnosis.

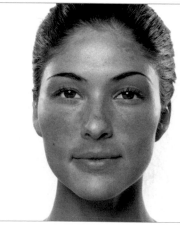

Melasma

ACNE

When it comes to acne, whether it appears, clears, worsens, or improves during pregnancy is completely unpredictable. In some cases the extra hormones promote a clear complexion while in others they cause a sudden flaring. If you find you are having problems with acne, consult your doctor for safe acne treatment during pregnancy. Topical treatments with antibiotics (clindamycin) and benzoyl peroxide are frequently prescribed.

How to Prevent and Treat Varicose Veins

- Get up and move around. Avoid standing or sitting for long periods of time. Walking helps the blood return to your heart.
- Always prop your feet up on a stool when sitting.
- Wear support stockings and start wearing them early, even in the first trimester of pregnancy, as a preventive measure.
- Sit with your legs higher than your head for at least half an hour a day.
- Avoid excessive weight gain.
- Avoid weight-bearing exercises.
- After you deliver and complete nursing, consider sclerotherapy injections, which are more effective than lasers. These injections, preformed by a dermatologist or vascular surgeon, can treat all vein sizes with a minimally invasive procedure that produces great results with very little scarring.

Other Pregnancy-Related Miscellaneous Annoyances

WHY ARE MY VEINS SHOWING?

Because of the added pressure caused by the increase in blood volume, veins pop out all over your body during pregnancy. Varicose veins are bulky blue/green veins on the inner thighs and back of the legs. Spider veins or telangiectasias are tiny purplish streaks that are most commonly seen on the outer thighs, ankles, and behind the knees, as well as on the face, neck, upper chest, and arms. In both cases, the vessels stretch as your body compensates for the extra blood flow that is going to your baby. With your pelvis engorged from the weight of the baby, more pressure is placed on your circulatory system.

Spider veins are not painful and usually disappear shortly after delivery. Varicose veins, on the other hand, can be quite unsightly and oftentimes downright painful. If you have a family history of varicose and spider veins, you will be predisposed to forming them during your pregnancy. However, you can take measures to prevent or decrease the symptoms (see box).

I HATE MY STRETCH MARKS!

Literally rips or microscars in the dermal layer of your skin, stretch marks, or striae, appear as skin is increasingly stretched during pregnancy. Initially surfacing as pinkish or reddish streaks running down your abdomen, breasts, hips, thighs, and even arms, they gradually fade to a lighter color. There is some evidence suggesting that susceptibility to stretch marks is hereditary. With almost 75%–90% of pregnant women experiencing them, stretch marks are one of the most talked about skin changes during pregnancy.

Unfortunately, you can't prevent stretch marks. No amount of cocoa butter, vitamin E, or alpha hydroxy acid will stop them from coming, and they can appear at any time during pregnancy—even on the day of delivery! Take comfort in knowing that these streaks will often fade to silvery white faint lines after delivery. Topical treatments such as Retin-A may help diminish their appearance and can be used following nursing. Newer laser treatments such as Fraxel and Thermage are also showing promise as permanent stretch mark remedies.

I HAVE A DRY, ITCHY ABDOMEN

As your beautiful belly grows, your skin stretches and tightens. This causes very uncomfortable dryness and itching. If you begin to experience severe itching late in your pregnancy, possibly accompanied by nausea, vomiting, loss of appetite, fatigue, and sometimes jaundice, you should contact your doctor. This could be a sign of cholestasis, which is related to the function of the liver. Your doctor may order blood tests to verify this diagnosis, which occurs in about one in every fifty pregnancies and resolves after pregnancy.

If the itching is intense and spreads to your arms and legs, it could be pruritic urticarial papules and plaques of pregnancy (PUPPP). PUPPP occurs in about one in every 150 pregnancies and is visible as itchy, reddish, raised patches on the skin that will go away after delivery.

To help alleviate your dry, itchy abdomen, keep your belly moisturized. Oatmeal-based moisturizers and oatmeal baths are excellent for itchy skin. You can also use products that contain alpha hydroxy acid, such as Amlactin, for more intense moisturization. Anti-itch products such as Sarna or calamine lotion may help relieve symptoms. Even applying an ice cube to a small itchy area can help relieve discomfort immediately. However, you should avoid scratching, which can tear and scar your skin. Your doctor will prescribe medications for both cholestasis and PUPPP.

HELP! I'M PLAGUED BY SKIN TAGS

Skin tags are very small loose growths of skin that usually appear under your arms and breasts and on your neck. They are caused by skin rubbing against skin in those locations. They are nothing to worry about and may disappear within six months of delivery. If they don't, see your dermatologist, as they can be easily removed with a quick in-office procedure.

Take No Chances

We're often asked whether various dermatological drugs or procedures are safe during pregnancy. Our response is generally this: it's always best to wait until after delivery and breastfeeding to start any kind of new treatment or medicine. Not only is the physiology of your body in a constant state of flux, but also the health and well-being of your baby are your first priority.

As with any other medical condition or concern that arises during pregnancy, talk to your obstetrician about changes in your skin that concern you. He or she has probably seen it before and will help you make the decisions that are best for both you and your baby.

> The Countdown

For some, the countdown doesn't stop once the baby arrives. Increased hair loss postpartum is normal. But how much is too much? Follow this easy test for one week to see whether you are losing more hair than normal.

STEP 1: Count and record the total number of hairs lost every day. Collect the hairs in your brush (be sure to start with a clean brush each day) and the hairs lost in the shower or wherever you find them. You can even put them in an envelope as you collect them throughout the day and count them at the day's end.

STEP 2: Repeat daily for one week.

STEP 3: At the end of your seventh day, add up the daily totals and divide by seven to get the average number of hairs lost per day.

If you are losing more than one hundred hairs per day on average, this may be a sign of telogen effluvium, or excessive shedding. Don't worry; you're not going bald. Telogen effluvium usually stops after a few weeks. If your hair shedding continues beyond that point, make an appointment with your doctor for a further evaluation.

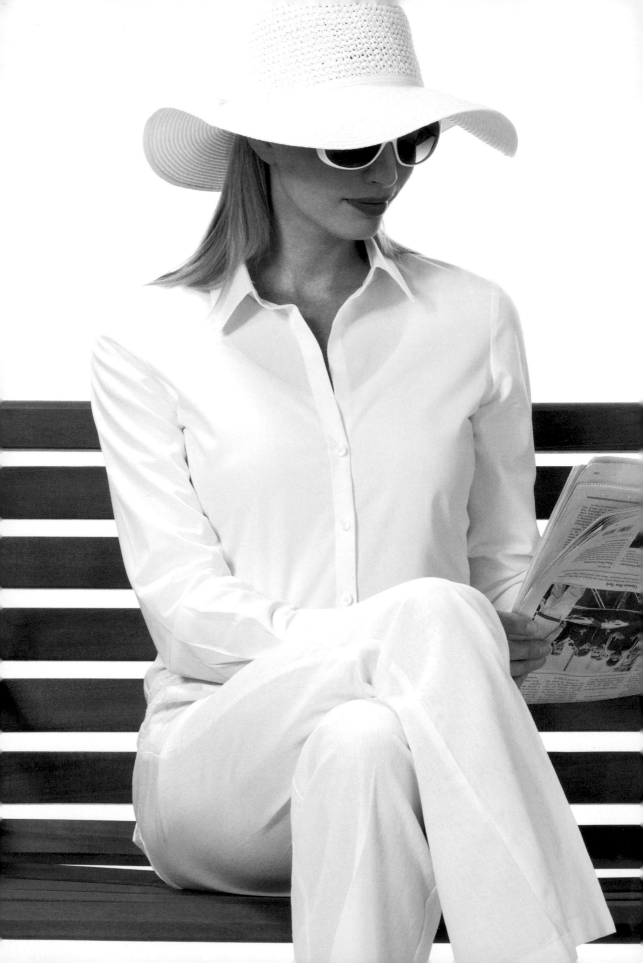

HERE COMES THE SUN

"Growing up through long, lousy winters in Illinois, my friends and I couldn't wait to get outside at the first sign of spring sun. We were desperate to get a tan, and we 'worked' at it with baby oil, reflectors—all the tools of the trade. But what we were really working at was burning our skin to a crisp and prematurely aging our skin."

Dr. Kathy Fields

There was a time not long ago when those with fair complexions went to great lengths to protect their skin from the sun. Pale, creamy skin was a symbol of wealth, whereas a brown, leathery complexion was a demonstrable stigma of the poor laboring working class. But early in the twentieth century, that all changed.

It was 1923 when fashion icon Coco Chanel was seen leaving Duke Wellington's yacht with a deep suntan after cruising from Paris to Cannes. Chanel inadvertently had gotten too much sun, but the press assumed the influential designer was making a fashion statement. Her bronzed skin was deemed the new status symbol—an emblem of leisure that came with affluence. Soon, women in Europe and America followed her lead, and the suntan came into vogue.

By the mid-1920s, "sun therapy" was being prescribed as a cure for everything from fatigue to tuberculosis. And because suntans hide a variety of ills, including acne, scars, cellulite, and spider veins, the trend never really faded, the way most tans and fads do.

We know significantly more about the sun's power and ability to harm our skin now than the medical community understood in the 1920s or even as recently as the 1970s, during our invincible teen years when sunscreens were not yet available to protect skin from the ravages of UV radiation. Yet the current widely publicized knowledge doesn't seem to stop today's young and beautiful from baring their bodies to catch a few rays. As the glamour of tanning persists, the rates of skin cancer in the United States continue to rise. And even more disturbing is the fact that, according to the National Cancer Institute, after years of increased sunscreen use, sunscreen protection has recently begun to decline.[1] We are seeing the devastating effects of the sun every day in our medical practices, from photoaged skin to melanomas.

Your brain is your best tool to prevent premature aging and the threats to your health and appearance posed by UV radiation. In this chapter, we'll explain the differences between the various ultraviolet rays, what they are doing to your skin, and how UV-induced changes reveal themselves over time. We'll share insights on selecting the most effective sun protection products and, importantly, using them correctly. And for those of you who are ready to commit to trading in your tan for healthier-looking skin, we'll share ways you can repair some of the signs of photoaging you may already have accumulated.

The ABCs of UV Radiation

The sun provides warmth, light, and life. It can also deliver blistering sunburns, premature aging, and skin cancer. In fact, during your lifetime, the sun showers literally tons of damaging photons onto your naked flesh.

The sun emits three kinds of UV light: long-wavelength UVA, medium-wavelength UVB, and short-wavelength UVC. The shorter the wavelength, the stronger the light. UVC radiation is absorbed by our atmosphere and never reaches the earth, which is a good thing because it has the strength to kill us instantly. On the other hand, the longer UVA and UVB rays do penetrate the atmosphere, and between the two they cause plenty of damage to our skin. As the ozone layer gets thinner, penetration by all wavelengths of UV light increases, resulting in earlier and more aggressive skin damage.

UVB, THE BURNING RAYS

We'll begin with UVB rays, which you are no doubt familiar with, as these are the rays that cause painful and visible sunburns. They're the ones your mother always warned you about because they're strongest between 10:00 a.m. and 2:00 p.m. during the summer months, when sunlight hits the earth more directly.

In the United States, the labeling of sunscreens, regulated by the FDA, is measured according to the SPF (sun protection factor) grading system. The SPF number refers to the product's ability to block out UVB radiation but does not pertain to the product's ability to block UVA light.

Along with burning (think *B* for "burn"), UVB rays can also cause skin cancer. The cancers associated with UVB radiation are most commonly the nonmelanoma types, basal cell and squamous cell carcinomas. These are the skin cancers that originate in the epidermis, the top layer of your skin, where the shorter UVB rays strike and cause damage. Because the burning effects of UVB radiation are so immediate and visible, not to mention painful, sunscreen technologies that protect us from UVB rays have advanced significantly since the late 1970s and are quite effective at blocking these rays.

UVA, THE AGING RAYS

UVA rays are commonly referred to as the "aging" rays (think *A* for "aging"). They are the long rays that penetrate deep into the dermis, causing tremendous damage over time. They have the ability to destroy our collagen and elastin, causing wrinkles and sagging. UVA rays also stimulate pigment-producing melanocytes to release brown melanin, resulting in "liver spots" on the face, hands, and chest—a true hallmark of aged skin. Persistent sun damage may eventually cause some of the pigment-producing cells to die, leaving white confetti-like spots technically known as guttate hypomelanosis on the skin. UVA rays further damage your RNA (ribonucleic acid), which is located in the cytoplasm of cells and contains the instructions for all the chemical reactions within the cell. This UVA damage compromises your body's ability to repair itself. And most problematically, UVA rays can mutate your DNA, eventually leading to skin cancer.

Often, the first sign of UVA damage appears in children. Those adorable freckles aren't quite so adorable when we understand they are a sign of skin injury in much the same way that an age spot is evidence of sun damage in an adult. People may claim they have always had freckles, but this is absolutely not true. No one is born with freckles. They are the body's response to sun damage, an indicator that you need to slather on broad-spectrum sunscreen or risk significant damage that will appear later in life.

UVA radiation is omnipresent. It strikes the earth and your skin from sunup to sundown, rain or shine, January through December. The rays are equally as strong at 7:00 a.m. as they are at noon and at 5:00 p.m. They are so powerful they can penetrate glass, some plastics, and clothing, especially loose cotton weaves and wet fabrics.

Unfortunately, most sunscreens available in the United States before the 1990s weren't created to block UVA radiation. UVA sunscreen agents used today include oxybenzophenone, zinc oxide, titanium dioxide, Mexoryl, and avobenzone. Each of these ingredients blocks UVA light to a greater or lesser degree. The most effective ones are zinc oxide, avobenzone, and Mexoryl.

What Are SPF and Broad-Spectrum, and Why Do We Need to Know?

Until June, 2011, the term SPF, or "sun protection factor," referred specifically to the level of UVB protection provided by your sunscreen. It was, and remains, a personal thing, meaning it's a rough estimate of the time you can spend in the sun before burning. For example, if you are light skinned and tend to burn in ten minutes on a summer day, applying a sunscreen with an SPF 15 will allow you to be in the sun fifteen times ten minutes (that's 150 minutes, or two and a half hours) before *burning*. Although SPF ratings will continue to be based on protection from UVB radiation, beginning in June, 2012, the addition of the term "broad-spectrum" will provide the

Can You Be Addicted to the Sun?

Yes! Some people actually have a real addiction to the pleasure of tanning. According to a study conducted by Dr. Anthony Liguori and published in the *Journal of the American Academy of Dermatology*, indoor tanning booths may be addictive.[2]

During a six-week period, a group of frequent tanning salon clients were offered three tanning sessions a week. Unbeknownst to them, some of the tanning beds emitted ultraviolet light and some did not. The participants consistently reported being in a better mood after having spent time in the UV bed, and when given a choice they invariably chose the bed emitting ultraviolet light. Most of the participants also said that if they went more than a few days without another tanning session, they would feel down.

The UV rays appear to trigger the release of endorphins—morphine-like substances in the brain that block pain and heighten pleasure—resulting in a natural "high." Just like smoking, this is a habit you will have to break if you want your skin to stand the test of time.

assurance that the sunscreen provides UVA protection that is proportionate to the level of UVB protection in that product.

Prior to the new FDA rules for sunscreen testing and labeling that were released in June, 2011, and required for all products marketed in the United Sates by December, 2012, there was no uniform system for measuring a sunscreen's ability to block UVA light. This meant that the term "broad-spectrum UVA/SPF sunscreen" could be misleading because it did not quantify the extent to which a particular product shielded against UVA damage. The FDA final rules on sunscreen efficacy testing and labeling are designed to address this. Read on.

The Paradox of Sunscreen

There is a phenomenon we call the "paradox of sunscreen" that pertains specifically to UVA light. In spite of the widespread use of sunscreen over the past thirty years, visible skin aging changes and skin cancer rates have continued to rise. If sunscreens were effectively protecting us, this would not be the case. The reason this paradox exists is the false sense of security people often get from using sunscreen. A high-SPF sunscreen might only prevent a UVB-induced sunburn, but a sunburn is nature's way of letting you know that you have had too much sun for your skin type and a signal that it is time to seek the shade. So, thanks to a product with an SPF 30, you might have spent three to four times longer in the sun, believing that you were protected. However, if your sunscreen blocked mainly UVB light and, to a much lesser extent, UVA light, you could easily have been exposed to three to four times more UVA light. Because UVA light is present in one-hundred-fold greater amounts in the environment than UVB light, the profound damage that is associated with UVA, i.e., aging and melanoma, has been on the rise.

The new sunscreen rules are designed to address the paradox of sunscreen with a new efficacy testing for "broad-spectrum" label claims. Beginning December, 2012, in order for a sunscreen to claim broad-spectrum activity, it must demonstrate effective UVA protection in proportion to its SPF claim. If a sunscreen does not pass the broad-spectrum test, it will be required to bear a

Stopping the Pain

We see two types of sunburns in our offices. First-degree burns are pink and swollen. Second-degree burns blister. We have two great tips to help relieve the pain and even stop the onset of the symptoms of sunburn:

1. If you suspect you have gotten too much sun and have an impending burn, take two aspirin immediately. Aspirin interrupts the inflammatory pathway that produces the signs and symptoms of a sunburn. So, with this advice, you may never see red or feel the pain. Always take aspirin with food and avoid it if you have a history of gastric ulcers or bleeding problems. ·

2. If it's already too late and your skin is inflamed, we recommend soaking pieces of cloth in whole milk and popping these compresses into the refrigerator or freezer. Once the cold milk compresses are ready, place them on your burned areas for twenty minutes. Keep trading them out for new ones as they warm up. The protein in the milk can be very effective for relieving the painful symptoms of a burn.

If you have a blistering burn, leave the blisters intact and see your dermatologist or physician. The blister acts as a natural Band-Aid. Once the blisters pop, cover the raw skin with an antibiotic ointment such as Polysporin to prevent infection.

warning that reads, "Skin cancer/skin aging alert: Spending time in the sun increases your risk of skin cancer and early skin aging. This product has been shown only to help prevent sunburn, not skin cancer or early aging."

The Funny Thing about Sunscreen

If you don't use it, it won't work. As obvious as this sounds, under-application of sunscreen is more the rule than the exception. When it comes to correct application of sunscreen, it is likely that the greater the SPF, the less you will apply. That's because higher protection levels tend to result in heavier, greasier or more whitening formulations, making compliance a problem. We recommend using a cosmetically elegant SPF 30 … broad-spectrum, of course … every day and reapplying it every few hours.

When sunscreen is applied correctly, SPF 15 blocks 93% of UVB rays; SPF 30 blocks 97% of UVB rays, and SPF 50 blocks 99% of UVB rays.

Invisible and Incidental Exposure to the Sun

One fallacy about sun exposure is that what you see is what you get. Unfortunately, sun protection is not that easy, and it's the stealth damage, in addition to the visible burns and tans, that leads to greater photoaging and cancer in the long run.

While most people know that skipping sunscreen when lounging at the pool is a bad idea, few realize that incidental sun exposure can be more damaging. Whether sitting in a sunny office, commuting on the freeway, or walking the dog, if we neglect to protect ourselves from daily sun damage, our skin will pay the price. And since 80% of the sun's rays penetrate clouds, you aren't safe on gloomy days either.

"Every day is sun-day according to your skin. Just twenty minutes of sun exposure a day adds up. Do the math and you'll see that this is equivalent to two straight weeks (that's fourteen eight-hour days) of exposure over the course of a year. You wouldn't spend two weeks baking in the sun without sunscreen, would you? This proves how important daily sun protection really is."

DR. KATIE RODAN

The collective damage associated with the sun may start to show on your skin by your twenties. Dermatologists once believed that 80% of a person's lifetime sun damage occurred by age eighteen. However, today there is good news. Recent medical studies have refuted this conventional wisdom and shown that only 20% of lifetime sun damage occurs by age twenty-three, with 10% accumulating per decade thereafter. So even if you were neglectful of sun protection as a child, you can make a huge difference in how you age going forward. It's never too late to start protecting yourself from the sun's rays.

Not All Skin Types Are Created Equal

Our skin color is the result of evolutionary changes that helped our ancestors survive and thrive in their environments. Fair skin evolved in northern climates such as Germany, Ireland, and Sweden. These regions distant from the equator lacked significant quantities of sunlight necessary for the skin to produce vitamin D, which is essential for bone calcification. By evolutionary design, fair skin allows better penetration of UVB radiation for the manufacturing of sufficient quantities of vitamin D at lower light levels. With less inherent sun protection, people with fair complexions who move to sunnier, warmer climates such as Florida are more prone to premature aging and skin cancer.

Darker-skinned individuals trace their ancestry to equatorial regions, where their deeper levels of melanin protected their skin from the DNA destruction associated with intense daily radiation. However, dark-complected individuals are not immune from sun-induced changes such as brown spots, melasma, and post-inflammatory hyperpigmentation. (Refer to Chapter Nine for more on hyperpigmentation.) In fact, the darker your natural skin color, the more likely you are to have cosmetic concerns related to hyperpigmentation. Although very dark black skin has a natural SPF of 13, dark-complected individuals still experience higher death rates than fair-skinned ones from skin cancer. We believe this occurs because skin cancer is less visible and therefore diagnosed later in dark-skinned people and is typically more aggressive, leading to an increased mortality rate. The important information to take away is that all skin types, dark and light, need protection from the sun to look good and stay healthy.

Sun Myths

It's important to be aware of the following myths:

MYTH: SUNSCREEN KEEPS YOU SAFE ALL DAY

Nothing can protect you 100% from UV rays, except sitting in a windowless room. Sunscreen is an important part of your defense against the sun, but you should consider other options such as UV-protective clothing, wide-brimmed hats, sunglasses, and ultimately staying out of the sun for the long-term benefit of your skin.

MYTH: THE SUN IS THE BEST SOURCE FOR VITAMIN D

There is an ongoing debate in the medical community that daily sun exposure is critical for production of adequate vitamin D. Vitamin D is a fat-soluble vitamin that prevents rickets in children, maintains bone density in adults, may inhibit certain cancers such as non-Hodgkin's lymphoma, and possibly lessens the risk of diseases such as multiple sclerosis. It is true that sunlight stimulates the production of vitamin D; however, the Skin Cancer Foundation recommends that you get your daily value of vitamin D from nonsun sources such as vitamin D–fortified milk, orange juice, salmon, and other fatty fishes or a multivitamin containing at least 1000 international units of vitamin D_3 daily.

MYTH: SUNBATHING IS A GOOD WAY TO CLEAR UP ACNE

People believe that sun helps to clear up their acne because a tan masks the redness of a breakout and may in fact dry pimples up a bit faster. However, over time, sun exposure causes breakouts rather than clears them. With every tan, cell turnover increases, building up more dead cells. As these dead cells pile up, pores become blocked, causing more breakouts. So, sunbathing is not a viable way to treat acne and will often make it worse. Check out our acne solutions in Chapter Eight for ways to manage acne-prone skin.

MYTH: SUNLESS TANNERS DARKEN SKIN, SO THEY PROTECT FROM SUNBURNS

Sunless tanners stain the color of your stratum corneum, which is the outermost layer of your skin. Suntans and sunburns affect the deepest layer of the epidermis, the stratum basale. These fake tans do not protect you from the sun.

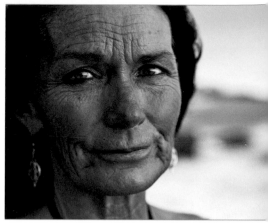

No number of birthdays can ever do this to your skin. This kind of aging comes only from exposure to uv light.

Photoaging and Photodamage

Photoaging and photodamage are two scientific terms for the same thing—the damage to skin caused by intense and chronic exposure to uv light.

uva light in particular is responsible for photoaging because it causes damage to both the epidermis and the

dermis. When uv rays from the sun or a tanning booth strike the skin, they initiate reactions, including inflammation, sunburn, and pigment cell activation, i.e., a tan. The uv rays also kill some cells and alter the DNA of others. Over time, with repeated exposure, collagen and elastin fibers break down, producing wrinkling and sagging. All these reactions working in unison result in premature aging and the formation of precancers and skin cancers.

Photodamage is cumulative, with sunscreen the one and only true sun damage prevention cream in existence today. Think of sunscreen as the best investment in your skin's future. Wearing it now can also save you thousands of dollars in corrective treatments later on.

Tiny Solar Scars Add up to Visible Wrinkles

uv irradiation damages and interferes with collagen production by producing enzymes called matrix metalloproteinases (MMPs). As these enzymes attack collagen fibers, the skin responds by attempting to heal the damage and in the process forms a "solar scar." With each dose of sunlight, the cycle continues, eventually creating a visible wrinkle. uv rays also break down elastin, the elastic fibers that keep skin resilient and able to bounce back after stretching. Hence, facial sagging occurs. As if wrinkling and sagging weren't enough, the crepey skin known to the dermatology trade as actinic elastosis on the side of the neck, the forearms, and backs of the hands is further evidence of photoaging.

Skin Cancer: The Sobering Facts

1.3 million people will be diagnosed with skin cancer this year.[3]

There are more new cases of skin cancer each year than breast, prostate, lung, and colon cancers combined.

The risk of developing melanoma, the most dangerous form of skin cancer, has more than doubled in the past decade. Yet melanoma is one of the easiest forms of cancer to prevent, and early detection and treatment are critical.

More than 90% of all skin cancers are caused by sun exposure, yet fewer than 33% of us routinely use sun protection.

Weakening of the Skin's Immune System

Sun compromises your skin's immune system by damaging Langerhans cells, the immune cells that live in the top layer of your skin. They are your body's first line of defense against the outside world. When the sun knocks these cells out, your immune system is temporarily knocked down. This can lead to a host of issues, including cold sores or fever blisters, but the problem can compound. With significant sun damage over time, your immune system becomes weakened and unable to ward off skin cancer.

Skin cancer is clearly the most devastating by-product of sun damage. Forty to fifty percent of Americans who live to age sixty-five will have skin cancer at least once. Outside of prevention, early detection is key for your health and possibly your survival. Because you look at your body every day, you have the ability to find suspicious spots well before you visit a doctor. In the following pages, we will share information about the three different types of skin cancer and how to identify each.

Skin Cancers

The three skin cancers caused by UV rays are as follows:

BASAL CELL CARCINOMA

This is by far the most common skin cancer, accounting for one million of the 1.3 million skin cancer diagnoses each year. Developing at the lowest level of the epidermis, this skin cancer often appears as a pink shiny bump on the top of the head, nose, face, neck, or chest. It doesn't hurt but may bleed and crust over. It is often mistaken for a pimple that doesn't heal because it just sits there and slowly grows. If you have something that resembles a pimple on your face for more than three months, it could be a cancer. Basal cell carcinoma seldom spreads to other parts of the body, but it can be disfiguring if not treated early.

> **? DID YOU KNOW**
>
> ONE BLISTERING CHILDHOOD SUNBURN CAN DOUBLE YOUR RISK OF DEVELOPING MELANOMA. SUNBURNS DAMAGE LANGERHANS CELLS, WHICH PROTECT YOUR IMMUNITY. ONE BAD BURN AS A CHILD CAN DAMAGE YOUR IMMUNE SYSTEM AND SET YOU UP FOR MELANOMA LATER IN LIFE.

SQUAMOUS CELL CARCINOMA

This skin cancer also develops in the uppermost layers of the epidermis. These red scaling patches that do not heal usually appear on areas of the body that have the most exposure to the sun such as your face, backs of hands, rims of ears, and lips. Squamous cell carcinoma is easy to treat in its early stages but if ignored can spread to other organs and even be fatal. Squamous cell carcinoma kills approximately 2,500 Americans each year.

The ABCDEs of Melanoma

Use these tips as a guideline to determine whether you may have melanoma.

A: Asymmetry—the spot isn't symmetrical and may have an odd shape

B: Border—look for a border that isn't sharp or defined

C: Color—the color is not uniform and may have different shades of red, brown, or black

D: Diameter—the spot is the size of a pencil eraser or larger

E: Evolution—the spot changes over time

MELANOMA

This is the deadliest skin cancer, although survival rates are improving. In 2003, approximately one-quarter of the people diagnosed with melanoma would die. Today that figure is one in seven, but the rate of melanoma continues to rise.

In 2007, the American Cancer Society estimated that the number of new melanoma cases was nearly 60,000. And in 2008, there were 62,480 new cases. A recent study reported in the January 2009 issue of the *Journal of Investigative Dermatology* looked at the data from 1992 to 2004 and found that rates of melanoma increased by 3.1 percent a year.[4] This aggressive growth rate is considered epidemic by some scientists.

People with light skin who spend a lot of time outdoors are at the highest risk, and three men are diagnosed with melanoma for every two women. The rationale is that men typically work outside more than women and that women are more inclined to use sun protection products when they are outside.

Although melanoma is associated with aging and sun exposure, it can develop at any time on anyone. Melanoma presents as a pigmented spot, and unlike basal cell and squamous cell carcinomas, it may appear in non-sun-exposed areas of the skin. Microscopically, melanoma starts in the lowest layers of the epidermis, expanding downward into the dermis, where it can metastasize through lymphatic and blood vessels, gaining access to the rest of the body and potentially becoming fatal. Early detection via a complete skin exam performed at least annually by a dermatologist is your best defense against this deadly foe.

"I found an old photo of my sister, my father, and me circa 1963 washing our 1960 Dodge Dart on a sunny day in Cleveland. Of note in the photo: the car was not equipped with seat belts, my father had a cigarette in his hand, and my sister and I both had golden brown suntans. No wonder the average life expectancy was almost ten years less back then."

LORI BUSH

Getting Checked for Skin Cancers

If you or your family has a history of skin cancer, we suggest you see your dermatologist at least once every six months for a skin check. There are also studies suggesting an increased risk of melanoma in people with a prior history of breast cancer or lymphoma. For fair-skinned individuals without any family history of skin cancer, we recommend seeing a dermatologist once per year. Be sure that your doctor does a thorough check of your entire body from head to toe, including your scalp, toes, and genitalia. It is also helpful if you can point out new or changing moles to your doctor.

Active Ingredients to Look for in Your Broad-Spectrum Sunscreen

To protect against UVA rays:

- Avobenzone (aka Parsol 1789): chemical block

- Mexoryl: chemical block

- Zinc oxide: inorganic

- Titanium Dioxide: inorganic

To protect against UVB rays:

- Octocrylene: chemical block

- Homosalate: chemical block

- Octisalate: chemical block

- Cinnamate: chemical block

- Ensulizole: chemical block

- Octinoxate: chemical block

- Padimate A: chemical block

- Padimate O: chemical block

Skin cancer is most common on the nose, but we also find malignant growths where people aren't as diligent about applying their sunscreen, particularly along the hairline, neck, ears, and upper torso. And between 5%–10% of all skin cancers develop on the eyelids, so wearing sunglasses is extremely important. Sunglasses will also protect you from cataracts and pterigiums, the little yellow bumps sometimes visible on the whites of your eyes.

DID YOU KNOW

FECAL MATTER MAY BE IN YOUR TANNING BED. A STUDY OF HIGHLY-RATED TANNING SALONS IN NEW YORK CITY FOUND TRACES OF FECAL MATTER AND OTHER BACTERIA THAT CAN LEAD TO INFECTIONS IN THE "SANITIZED" BEDS. JUST ANOTHER DANGER OF INDOOR TANNING.[6]

The Facts about Sunless Tanning

In spite of all of the education and warnings and much to our chagrin, many people still devote time to working on their tans. Some are convinced they look and feel healthier, skinnier, and sexier with a tan. There are several popular ways people get that "sun-kissed glow" without setting foot outdoors, and unfortunately, they aren't all entirely safe.

TANNING SALONS

If you think a tanning bed is a safe alternative to the sun, think again. While the tanning industry is happy to have you know they filter out most of the UVB burning rays, the reality is that sun lamps emit significantly greater quantities of UVA, contributing to premature skin aging and increasing the incidence of both melanoma and nonmelanoma skin cancers. Nonetheless, tanning salons are extremely popular. About twenty-eight million Americans visit a tanning salon at least once a year, and nearly two and a half million of those visitors are teens. Because the industry is unregulated, tanning salons in most states allow minors under the age of eighteen to use the tanning beds without parental consent. However, we know that UV radiation causes skin cancer at a young age and may be the reason melanoma is the most common cancer killing people in their twenties. In fact, the World Health Organization classifies UV tanning beds as "carcinogenic to humans," their highest cancer risk category.[5]

SPRAY-ON TAN SALONS

We are wary of spray-on sunless tanning booths. The active ingredient in self-tanners is dihydroxy-acetone (DHA), a color additive used to stain human skin. The fine mist delivery of DHA is easily inhaled during application in spray booths. Some research has shown this method of application can result in DHA entering the bloodstream via the lungs. Since no thorough studies have been

Sunscreen: A Little Dab Won't Do Ya

Sunscreen manufacturers determine SPF in a laboratory setting. Subjects put on a certain amount of sunscreen per centimeter of skin and are then exposed to a solar simulator (a lamp that creates UV radiation similar to sunlight). The amount of sunscreen applied for this test is quite heavy, far more than most people ever use at the beach.

The reality is that an SPF 80 can act like an SPF 3 if you only apply a thin layer. Therefore, we urge patients to layer their sunscreen. Apply your sunscreen thirty minutes before exposing yourself to the sun. Let it dry down for at least fifteen minutes and then reapply another coat just before your tennis match, mountain hike, or other outdoor activity. That way, you'll have a fighting chance of achieving the full SPF rating and maximizing the potential UVA protection of your product.

completed on the systemic effects of DHA toxicity, we cannot confidently recommend this sunless-tanning method, and we're not the only ones concerned: the FDA has issued an advisory cautioning consumers against "unwanted exposure to DHA." Until the effects of DHA absorption are known, we recommend limiting your use of sunless tanning booths to special occasions only.

SELF-TANNERS

Getting your glow from a bottle, tube, or handheld spray is the safest way to simulate a tan. Because this is what we do, we'd like to share our tips. First, take a shower and exfoliate every part of your body where you will be applying the self-tanner. Next, use a heavy cream-based moisturizer on your knees, elbows, toes, toenails, heels, and ankles to prevent the self-tanner from concentrating in those areas where the stratum corneum is thickest. To avoid orange palms, use protective gloves and apply the sunless tanner very quickly. We prefer a foam-based self-tanner for a more even application. Use an old washcloth and lightly blend in any excess to avoid streaks. Acetone or nail polish remover can be used to remove streaks if you make a mistake.

If you find it difficult to obtain a uniform color from these products, try moisturizers that contain low concentrations of DHA. Their daily application hydrates your skin while color gradually builds.

Undoing What's Done

Because so much environmental aging is the result of exposure to the UV radiation epidemic in the United States, several chapters in this book are dedicated to helping reverse the effects of past sun sins. This is one place where a spoonful of vanity goes a long way.

As dermatologists, we see it as our primary responsibility to protect and preserve skin's health. However, even after years of preaching and cutting skin cancers off peoples' bodies, many still don't heed our advice.

Once somebody has invested hundreds, even thousands, of dollars to correct the cosmetic effects of sun damage, sun protection is another story. So if you find the dreaded wrinkle creates greater motivation to use sunscreen than the fear of skin cancer, so be it. You'll still have healthier skin in the end, and that's what we care about most.

Selecting Sunscreens

Avobenzone, zinc oxide, or Mexoryl, broad-spectrum sunscreens that block both UVA and UVB rays, are essential. Many sunscreens today are also fortified with active cosmetic ingredients, from vitamin C and E to broccoli and green tea, that may help prevent free radical damage. These anti-

Barbie and Social Responsibility

Back in 1971, Malibu Barbie was teaching our young daughters that sporting a suntan was groovy. Roll the clock forward to the new millennium and Malibu Barbie comes with her own miniature bottle of sunscreen, SPF 60. She still has a tan, however, which leads us to ask, "where's the sunless tanner?" Maybe she left it in the Barbie Dream Car.

oxidants may very well make a difference, so we encourage people to hedge their bets and select sunscreens containing antioxidants.

Make sure you are investing in a sunscreen that is going to provide you with broad-spectrum UVA and UVB protection. Not all sunscreens are created equal. We encourage you to check the active ingredients label on the back of the box or tube to be certain you are getting safe and effective protection.

Two kinds of sunscreen blockers protect against UV rays: physical and chemical. Physical blockers include ingredients such as zinc oxide, which you may remember as the white paste lifeguards often wear on their noses. Physical blockers do exactly what their name implies—they physically block or reflect the ultraviolet rays back into the environment, thereby protecting the skin's surface. Zinc oxide is an effective ingredient that doesn't tend to irritate skin. Today, cosmetically elegant forms of zinc oxide exist that appear transparent and are less whitening. Zinc is a great option for people with rosacea because it reduces the appearance of redness.

Chemical blockers include ingredients such as avobenzone (Parsol 1789) or Mexoryl. These ingredients have been approved by the FDA and, in addition to zinc oxide, offer the best protection available today against damaging UVA rays. While effective, avobenzone can break down in the presence of sunlight ... problematic for a sunscreen. Thankfully, there are advances in skincare technology that do double duty, improving the quality of your skin as they protect avobenzone. Look for facial sunscreens that include colorless carotenoids, our favorite multi-tasking avobenzone stabilizer.

Finally, although we love makeup with sunscreen, it generally doesn't sufficiently protect your skin. Use your broad-spectrum sunscreen first and then apply your makeup with SPF for added protection.

Is Your Cell Phone Wearing Your Sunscreen?

Apply your sunscreen every day, at least a half hour before you go out into the sun, so it has time to penetrate and completely dry on the surface of your skin. Sunlight, sweat, and water degrade the efficacy of sunscreen ingredients, so it's important to reapply every two hours to maintain the level of protection you need. Even if you are just heading to work in an office building, sunscreen won't stay with you all day. Your phone will collect sunscreen, as will your hands, lunch napkins, and anything else that rubs up against your face. You should get in the habit of reapplying a broad-spectrum sunscreen before you get in the car, especially if you are going to be stuck in traffic. And don't forget to apply sunscreen to the tops of your hands. We can easily tell the difference between a frequent driver and a frequent passenger, because the aging characteristics appear on the side of the body closest to the window.

In addition, apply sunscreen liberally. One full ounce should be adequate to cover your entire body. If you're not sure what an ounce looks like, visualize a shot glass. You will need a teaspoon to cover your entire face. A teaspoon is roughly equivalent to the size of a quarter. If you apply your

Although efforts to protect skin from the ravages of the sun literally date back to the ancient Egyptians, the first commercial attempts to produce sunscreen took place in the 1930s. One of the first sunscreens was formulated by chemist Franz Greiter who was inspired by a painful sunburn he experienced on Piz Buin mountain in the Swiss Alps. His SPF 2 sunscreen was eventually marketed by a company bearing the name of the Swiss mountain where he was sunburned. The Piz Buin sunscreens are still available in Europe to this very day ... allbeit with more adequate levels of SPF protection.

sunscreen properly over your entire body, you personally should polish off a bottle during your weekend at the beach. While this may seem expensive, it's an investment that will pay dividends for years to come.

Finally, watch the expiration date. Like all good cosmetics and medicines, the fresher the ingredients, the more effective the product. Additionally, if you keep your sunscreen out in the sun (such as on a beach towel) or in the glove compartment of your car, the heat may cause the active ingredients to break down, which means the sunscreens may not be as effective. Look for signs of formula breakdown such as color change, watery separation, or change in consistency. If these occur, throw the damaged bottle out and purchase a new one.

Additional Skin Protection Tips

These additional tips will help keep your skin looking great:

WEAR CLOTHING

The sun is a lot more powerful than a little blob of sunscreen. Donning a wide-brimmed hat and protective clothing can help further safeguard your skin. And we don't mean just a simple visor or baseball cap, because those really provide only enough shade to cover a small strip down the center of your face. When it comes to clothing, a sheer T-shirt is not enough to protect your body either. In general, the denser the fabric, the better the protection, so a long-sleeved nontransparent shirt will protect you better than a short-sleeved thin cotton top. A typical cotton T-shirt has an SPF of only about seven, and when it is wet, this decreases to an SPF of three to four. Therefore, we suggest giving your clothes a valuable fashion test: hold your shirt up to the sun. If you can see through it, you need a thicker material to protect your skin. To fortify your clothing, consider treating it with a laundry additive such as Rit Sun Guard to enhance the UV-guarding capabilities.

USE AN UMBRELLA

We have many patients who stand around at their kids' sporting events in the blazing sun for hours. We can't stress how important it is to get out of the direct sunlight. Soccer moms, don't sacrifice your skin. Instead, start an umbrella trend in your community.

INVEST IN UV SHIELDS FOR YOUR CAR

UV shields can be adhered to the window to provide some protection. Better still, have the car manufacturer tint your windows. The percentage of tint is regulated in most states. A higher percent tint might be allowed if you have a note from your doctor stating you're at risk for skin cancer.

USE YOUR BLINDS

If you sit by a window in your office, use the blinds. Remember that UVA rays penetrate glass and some plastic. We absolutely advocate pulling down the shade when you are in an airplane. You are high up in the atmosphere where the sun's rays are unfiltered, rendering them many-fold stronger.

WEAR A UV WRISTBAND

There are UV Sensitive Wristbands that change color when you are exposed to UV light. This is a great reminder of the incidental sun exposure you receive throughout the day.

A Final Word on Sunscreen

If we haven't convinced you to use sunscreen because it can protect you from painful sunburns, reduce the impact of aging, and help prevent skin cancers, consider the fact that studies show protected skin is better able to repair itself. Sun protection is the single most important way to keep your skin young and healthy looking. But don't despair if you have a history of basking in the sun. We grew up in the 1970s before sunscreen was around, spending every available opportunity trying to get a tan. Take solace in the fact that there are many options to protect yourself today and plenty of techniques to reduce the appearance of photoaging. Start by using your sunscreen every day. Your skin will thank you for it, and it may save your life.

Check Yourself with a Skin Cancer Self-Exam[7]

Do more than just powder your nose in the bathroom. Take a few minutes to thoroughly check the spots on your body. Refer back to the ABCDEs of melanoma for tips on finding cancerous spots. And remember: early detection is key! Do this exam at least once per year, recording any spots you find and especially ones that change in size, shape, or color. Make sure to notify your dermatologist of anything that looks suspicious.

STEP 1: Undress and stand in front of a mirror. Lift your arms above your head and examine your whole body—front, back, and both sides.

STEP 2: Take a closer look. Bending your elbows, study your forearms, the backs of your upper arms, and your palms.

STEP 3: Next, look at the backs of your legs and feet. Pay attention to detail—look in between your toes and on the soles of your feet.

STEP 4: Using an additional hand mirror, look at the back of your neck and scalp. Don't forget to part your hair different ways, looking for bumps in all possible locations.

STEP 5: Last but definitely not least, use an additional hand mirror to check your back and buttocks.

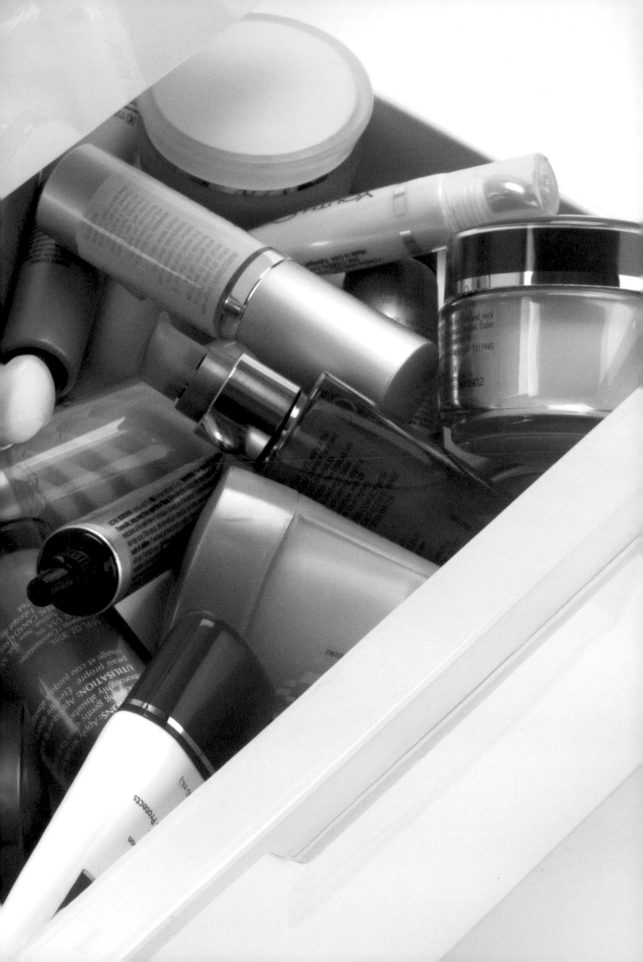

RAISE YOUR EXPECTATIONS

"Moisturizers can be like the 'emperor's new clothes.' So often
we have met patients who are willing to spend hundreds
of dollars on products without scientific proof of efficacy,
satisfied that their wrinkles 'look a little less noticeable.'
We tell them to expect more!"

Dr. Katie Rodan

How do you choose your skincare products? Are your selections based on a consultation from a dermatologist or a recommendation from a friend, or are they Oprah's favorites? For most people, regular visits to a dermatologist are neither practical nor feasible, so many turn to a skincare maven friend or a cosmetic salesperson for advice. While this may be an okay place to start, we want to offer our expertise to help make you a skincare expert yourself.

Desperately Seeking Benefits

With all the advancements made in skincare technology over the past two decades, we find that women continue to have very low expectations when it comes to achieving real, visible results from their pricey products. We observe that many of the benefits are more experiential or psychological than clinical or physiological. And that's no surprise. From the cosmetic counter consultation and the indulgent textures and fragrances to the etched glass jar that tells you "You're worth it," the multibillion-dollar beauty industry knows how to create a very seductive experience indeed. Even products with labels that sport a heady, scientific lexicon of new "breakthrough" ingredient names frequently disappoint in their ability to deliver visible results.

On the other hand, as dermatologists and as skincare consumers, we know there are real benefits to be derived from the science of credible companies in the skincare industry. We've seen ingredient and formulation advancements that make affordable skincare, especially for the treatment of common dermatology concerns, accessible to everyone. So if your drawerful of rejected skincare potions has you believing that you just have to live with less than a clear, radiant complexion, we've got great news. There's no need to resign yourself to covering flaws with makeup, resorting to plastic surgery, or just accepting the inevitable. With a little "industry insider" perspective and a bit of patience, we're confident you can find the right products and daily regimen to give you the impressive results that today's advanced formulations are often capable of delivering.

Are you confused about what is right for you when you approach that "wall of skincare" at the drugstore? If so, you're not alone. You may observe what merchandising experts using hidden cameras have captured—the skincare aisle can be a very confusing and intimidating place. In fact, when overwhelmed by an abundance of choice, many people walk away. In his 2004 book, *The Paradox of Choice*, Barry Schwartz provides strong evidence supporting his theory that the fear of making the wrong decision often leads to no product being purchased at all.

Because we know the right at-home program can make a tremendous difference in your skin's appearance, we want to raise your expectations for what your skincare can deliver. By helping you prioritize your issues, analyze your skin, and use the right products and treatments, we are confident we can prove to you that your skin can look better today than it did even ten years ago. However, it is important to remember that although it may be easy to make broad, sweeping statements about what a good skincare program should consist of, as dermatologists we know that skincare is not about generalities but about treating your individual needs. Lists of products that "everyone needs" probably won't address your particular concerns because there is no "one-size-fits-all" solution to skin.

Be Your Own Dermatologist

To achieve the clear, glowing skin you desire, you need to analyze your individual needs and treat your face as a whole. We want to teach you to look at your face the way we do and become your own dermatologist of sorts. We don't recommend that you sit in front of an 8x makeup mirror every day, torturing yourself with excessive magnification. Instead, as the needs of your skin change, we'd like you to become more observant and a little more obsessive about your skin. To remind yourself of your top concerns, refer to the workbook page in Chapter One.

Once you have determined what your goals and needs are, take a look at how you care for your skin. Is your routine consistent? What should stay, what needs to go, and what should change completely to create your individual program?

The program you adopt may consist of lifestyle changes, a targeted at-home skincare regimen, and possibly dermatologist-administered procedures that address issues topical products cannot.

What's a Neuropeptide Anyway?

True confession: even as ingredient-savvy dermatologists, we are sometimes baffled by all the fancy fabricated names that are designed to make cosmetics sound like drugs and make ordinary moisturizers sound like breakthrough treatments. Therefore, we do what you should do: we look at the ingredient declaration list for the standardized information about what is really in the product. In the United States, INCI names (International Nomenclature of Cosmetics Ingredients) are mandated as part of the labeling of all skincare products. And while the formulation, or recipe, for how these ingredients are put together can impact the safety and efficacy of these ingredients, understanding what is actually in the product is a good place to start.

But no matter how much we study a label or do our research to select a product, there is always a chance the product will not work or, worse yet, cause an undesirable reaction. If you purchase a product that does not meet your expectations, we encourage you to contact the manufacturer. The most reputable manufacturers want to ensure you have a good experience and will provide advice on how to use the product for optimal results, exchange the product for one that may be better for your skin's needs, or refund your money when you aren't satisfied.

⊕ Who's Watching Out for You?

You should take heart in knowing there are regulatory agencies protecting you as a consumer of skincare products, but that doesn't necessarily obviate the adage "Caveat emptor," or "Let the buyer beware."

The NAD (National Advertising Division) of the Council of Better Business Bureaus is the advertising industry's self-regulation forum for truth in advertising. In the competitive beauty industry, companies monitor each other, calling misleading claims to the attention of this agency. Beyond the industry's self-governing practices, the FTC (Federal Trade Commission) oversees laws created to protect consumers from untruthful and deceptive advertising. It is important to understand that larger companies are on the radar of these regulatory agencies and therefore tend to be more conservative in their claims. By the same token, consumers should be aware that some small niche companies may go unnoticed by these agencies, pushing the limit by making unlawful product claims.

In terms of oversight of products themselves, the FDA regulates "OTC" (over-the-counter) and prescription drugs for labeling and safety requirements but does not generally regulate cosmetic products or cosmetic ingredients. However, the FDA will intervene when a cosmetic product makes claims that are deemed drug claims by FDA guidelines.

Because cosmetics are less regulated than pharmaceuticals, the cosmetics industry has created a self-governing organization called the Personal Care Products Council (PCPC, formerly known as Cosmetics, Toiletries and Fragrance Association). By visiting www.cosmeticsinfo.org, you can get safety and efficacy information about cosmetics ingredients and other factual information from the industry's consumer advocates.

What's a Drug Facts Box?

A clue to the consumer: in the United States, if there is a "drug facts" label on the package or insert and the ingredient list separates and calls out an "active ingredient," it is an OTC drug. An ingredient cannot be listed as an "active ingredient" on a purely cosmetic product.

Active Ingredient: only ingredients regulated by FDA as drugs may be listed here

Purpose: tells you the condition for which this product is regulated by the FDA

Uses: this section contains the specific regulated usage information

Warnings: listed here are any known possible contraindications or adverse effects of the product; this information is required on all drugs but not on cosmetics

Directions: this tells you the recommended manner in which you should use the product

Inactive ingredients: this contains the other ingredients in the product that are not regulated as drugs; these ingredients may provide other cosmetic benefits not indicated under "uses"

Drug Facts

Active ingredient	Purpose
Salicylic Acid (2%)	Acne medication

Uses
• For the treatment of acne

Warnings
For external use only

When using this product
• Using other topical acne medications at the same time or immediately following use of this product may increase dryness or irritation of the skin. If this occurs, only one medication should be used unless directed by a doctor.
• Do not get into eyes. If excessive skin irritation develops or increases, discontinue use and consult a doctor.
• Apply to affected areas only.
• Do not use on broken skin or apply to large areas of the body.

Keep out of reach of children. If swallowed, get medical help or contact a Poison Control Center immediately. Avoid contact with eyes. If contact occurs, flush thoroughly with water.

Directions
• Wet skin and massage evenly onto skin and back.
• Rinse off and pat dry.
• Avoid contact with eyes.

Inactive ingredients
water, polyethylene, ammonium laureth sulfate, diethylhexyl sebacate, butylene glycol, allyl methacrylates crosspolymer, hydroxyethyl acrylate/sodium acryloyldimethyl taurate copolymer, cetearyl alcohol, magnesium aluminum silicate, squalane, polygonum cuspidatum root extract, allantoin, ceteareth-20, sea whip extract, yeast extract, sucrose, bis-behenyl/isostearyl/phytosteryl/dimer dilinoleyl dimer dilinoleate, caprylic/capric triglyceride, glyceryl stearate, PEG-100 stearate, polysorbate 60, dehydroxanthan gum, sodium salicylate, fragrance, disodium EDTA, methylchloroisothiazolinone, methylisothiazolinone, potassium sorbate, phenoxyethanol [iln32847]

SAMPLE DRUG FACTS BOX

Answering Common Product-Related Questions

Needless to say, when it comes to making the best skincare selections and achieving the best outcomes, you need to be armed with the best information. Although we can't anticipate them all, below are answers to some of the most common questions we hear from our patients.

Q. Aren't all cleansers the same? Can't I just use any soap and then spend my money on other, more important, products?

A. Your cleanser may be your most important product choice because cleansing is not a generic, one-size-fits-all process and matching your cleanser appropriately to your needs affects everything that happens afterward. Cleansers are not only meant to remove makeup, dirt, and grime but also should prepare your skin for the next step in your program. And because the act of cleansing can disrupt the skin's fragile moisture barrier, if you choose the wrong cleanser, you may be setting your skin up for future irritation.

When looking for a cleanser, you should make it simple—identify your most important skincare issue and find a cleanser that addresses that concern. For instance, if you have acne or are acne prone, look for a cleanser that is medicated with an antiacne ingredient. And for more oily skin, a bubbly surfactant-based cleanser will do a good job. If you are treating skin dullness or discolorations, exfoliation at least once a day as part of your cleansing routine will help brighten skin and enable medications and active cosmetic ingredients to better penetrate. And if you have sensitive skin, look for a creamy, fragrance-free cleanser that does not leave your skin feeling dry and tight once you rinse it off.

Many of us have been conditioned to believe that we need a cleanser to foam up with lots of suds to effectively clean our skin. However, suds are not always necessary and are oftentimes undesirable. (Just think about what happens when you put foaming dishwashing liquid in your dishwasher—you mop up suds for hours.)

When it comes to facial cleansers, gel cleansers that foam are often too harsh for many skin types. Surfactants that generate copious foam tend to be more irritating for those with dry or sensitive skin, although they are often well tolerated and preferred by those with very oily skin.

Most of us need to be careful not to strip too many lipids from our skin, as this causes disruption of the moisture barrier and leads to chronic low-grade inflammation that causes skin to look dull and more aged. Rule of thumb: the amount of cleansing suds should decrease as skin becomes dryer or more sensitive.

In general, remember that "squeaky clean" may be desirable for your dishes but not for your skin. Overcleansing can actually strip away your lipid barrier, making skin more susceptible to irritation. As an overall tip, we recommend that you use a soap-free cleanser, formulated specifically for the face.

Q. What happens when the wrong products are used together? Can I tell whether they are incompatible?

A. Unfortunately, when you purchase a product, you often don't receive information on how it will interact with other products you may be using. And if you combine incompatible products, there's a high likelihood you won't get the benefits you want. Sometimes the ingredients in different products counteract each other, so you simply won't experience the intended benefits of either product. Or, conversely, you may experience tandem irritation. This means that if you were to use either of the products independently, your skin would be fine, but when you use them together, your skin experiences irritation. Third, you may experience "product incompatibility," which you can easily test for by rubbing your face after the product has dried. If it peels, balls, or curdles, there is product incompatibility. The lesson is that in order to get the most from your skincare, you should develop a regimen that works compatibly or even synergistically to deliver measurable results.

The order in which you use products can also be important. One product may create an environment on your skin that enhances penetration of subsequent products, while another may actually block products or ingredients from penetrating the skin. Rule of thumb: after cleansing (and toning, if indicated), use liquids and/or serums first, then gels, then lotions, and then creams or balms. Simply stated, when layering products, go from the thinnest formulation to the thickest.

Q. How can I tell whether my skin is sensitive to a product before I cause my whole face to rebel?

A. Whenever you have concerns that you may be sensitive to a product, simply administer a "home patch test." Before you begin using the product on your face, start with a test on your neck. This is a good indicator of a potential facial reaction, and any reaction on your neck will be less visible than testing on your face. Apply the product to a small area on the side of your neck three times a day for three to four days. If you find that your skin reacts, return the product to the manufacturer. Most reputable manufacturers will be happy to refund your money or provide an exchange product that will be more compatible with your skin type.

Also note that sometimes a reaction doesn't necessarily mean you should write off the ingredient entirely. It may just be the concentration of an ingredient or the way a product is formulated that is causing your reaction. For instance, your skin may react negatively to benzoyl peroxide at 10%, but at 2.5% it may work well to treat your acne without causing any irritation.

Face Wash 101

There are ideal methods to everything, basic skincare included:

- Skip the soap. Instead, choose a cleanser that's right for your skin type.

- Remove long-wearing makeup first.

- Avoid washcloths because they can be too aggressive on skin. Instead, use fingertips to apply cleanser in gentle, circular movements.

- Rinse thoroughly with warm—not hot—water.

- Use only clean towels to dry your skin to avoid bacterial contamination.

Myth: Splashing cold water on skin after cleansing closes pores. **Fact:** Remember that pores don't have trap doors that open and close, so water temperature won't affect the size of your pores.

Q. Is it possible for my skin to become "used to a product" and not respond anymore?

A. If you start to no longer see the results that your product was once delivering, there are several possible reasons why. In some cases, the ingredient may stop working for you because of changes in your skin's needs or the climate you're living in. If you think this is the case, take a break for a bit and then try it again after a few weeks. Or, more often, your skincare problem has escalated in severity and requires a stronger medicine to treat it properly. Another possibility is that your skin has achieved its maximum benefit and that you are basically in a "maintenance mode." In this case, even though you're not noticing daily improvement, your skin is still benefiting from the treatment.

Q. When I start a new skincare regimen that contains active ingredients, what should I expect during the crossover process? Will my skin get worse before it gets better? Will I get used to the irritation? How long should I give a product before I give up on it?

A. The more active the ingredients or the more intense the exfoliation in the skincare regimen, the more likely you are to go through an adjustment period. Your skin is an amazing organ, however—it is very adaptable and will usually adjust to new products within a few days, though in some cases with strong medicines such as Retin-A that can cause peeling and redness, it may take weeks or even months for your skin to go through this "accommodation" process.

Our advice is to take it slow. When starting a medicated regimen, you may want to begin using a product once every other day. If you see that your skin is starting to get flaky, dry, irritated, or sensitive, take a break for a few days and use a very gentle product without any active ingredients and allow your skin to normalize. Then you can start using the active product again. And try to be patient. If we were treating you in our offices, we'd ask you to come back in two months to check your progress, so give a product containing medicines sixty days to achieve significant improvement. Contrary to popular belief, even if your skin responds to a new medication or treatment with some stinging or flaking, it should not be making the problem worse, which is a complaint with certain acne medicines. This is a common misconception. More likely than not, as you initiate a therapeutic program, you are more in tune with your skin, paying closer attention to everything that happens. So if you have a hormone surge that causes the acne to flare, you blame it on the treatment.

However, if a product is causing burning, swelling, and itching that worsens with each product usage, this could mean you are allergic to one of the ingredients and must stop using the product immediately. If you suspect an ingredient allergy, we recommend seeing a dermatologist for patch testing to determine what the ingredient is, as you will likely encounter it in other products as well.

Q. If my product contains a particular ingredient, does it mean I can be sure it will deliver the results I've heard about?

A. Not necessarily. For an ingredient to be effective in a product, it must be used at clinically effective levels. Sometimes ingredients are formulated only for "label claims," meaning the product contains the ingredient but not at the level that has been proven effective. For OTC products, an active ingredient must be used within an FDA-approved range, but this is not the case for active cosmetic ingredients such as peptides and retinoids. While it may be difficult to determine whether there is a sufficient level of an ingredient in the product to be efficacious, watch out for products that advertise the benefits of the ingredient rather than the benefits of the total product. In virtually all cases, it is about not just the ingredient but rather the ingredient, the application, and the formulation.

What's the Difference between Drugs, Cosmetics, and "Cosmeceuticals"?

When it comes to skincare products, knowing what you're really getting can be more difficult than you might expect. What makes one product a medicine, another a cosmetic, and another a "cosmeceutical"? According to the FDA, "The difference between a cosmetic and a drug is determined by a product's intended use."[1] A drug quite simply changes the structure and function of the skin while treating a specific problem.

But even this FDA explanation may not help you sort through the complicated regulatory systems. For instance, a shampoo is intended for cleansing the hair, and this would put it into a cosmetic category. However, if a shampoo is formulated to contain an OTC or a prescription drug at an effective level, even though the intended use is still as a shampoo, the shampoo is considered a treatment for dandruff, seborrheic dermatitis, or psoriasis and therefore is a drug.

To further confuse the matter, active drug ingredients such as salicylic acid may go into products at lower concentrations, rendering the product a cosmetic, not a drug. So at the end of the day, it's a combination of the ingredient, the concentration, the claims, and the intended use that determines what category a product falls into.

With certain ingredients, no matter what the concentration, the product is considered a drug. For instance, an antidandruff shampoo that contains ketoconazole will be labeled as a drug. At a concentration of 1% it will be labeled with a drug facts box as an OTC product, but at a concentration of 2%, it is an Rx drug and will require a prescription. Very confusing indeed.

To help you understand your products on the most basic level, we've provided these simple definitions of a prescription drug, OTC drug, cosmetic, and cosmeceutical:

PRESCRIPTION DRUGS

As defined by the FDA, a drug is: 1. A substance intended for use in the diagnosis, cure, mitigation, treatment, or prevention of disease. 2. A substance (other than food) intended to affect the structure or any function of the body. Regulated by the FDA, prescription drugs are available only by prescription from a physician. To be considered a drug, they have gone through a New Drug Application (NDA), an Amended New Drug Application (ANDA), or a Supplemental New Drug Application (SNDA). Retinoic acid or tretinoin, which people know by the brand names Retin-A or Renova, is an example of a prescription-regulated drug that is commonly used for its aesthetic benefits.

How Can You Tell Whether Your Skincare Is Working?

If you really want proof that your product is making a difference for your skin, you can do what we do during our product development process: conduct some clinical testing on yourself. Use your usual routine on one side of your face and your new program or product on the other side. Do this for a few weeks and see which side of your face looks and feels better. Then get another opinion. We use trained clinical investigators, but you can get a "blind" opinion from your spouse or best friend by not revealing which side is receiving the new product.

Keep in mind that just because your product is positioned in an attractive subcategory, be it herbal, organic, dermatologist-developed, etc., doesn't mean it's necessarily superior or right for you. You should still expect the product to deliver on its promise.

? DID YOU KNOW?

MANY MEDICINES IN PRESCRIPTION DRUGS ARE ALSO AVAILABLE IN OVER-THE-COUNTER PRODUCTS THAT DO NOT REQUIRE A PRESCRIPTION.

OVER-THE-COUNTER (OTC) DRUGS

The FDA defines OTC drugs as safe and effective for use by the general public without a doctor's prescription. The same ingredient that is in a prescription drug may also be available in an OTC product, depending on the concentration. However, some OTCs are not available by prescription. If a cosmetic claims that it has an active ingredient, it must contain an OTC medicine and will have a drug facts box on the label. Examples of OTCs are products with salicylic acid or dimethicone making claims for treating specific conditions under the guidelines and regulations of the USFDA OTC Monograph system. Additionally, in the United States, sunscreens are regulated as OTC drugs.

COSMETICS

According to the FDA, cosmetics are "articles intended to be rubbed, poured, sprinkled, or sprayed on, introduced into, or otherwise applied to the human body... for cleansing, beautifying, promoting attractiveness, or altering the appearance." Cosmetics are available without a prescription and affect only the epidermal or more superficial layers of the skin. They do not change the form and function of the skin. For example, hyaluronic acid, shea butter, and glycerin are ingredients that may be found in cosmetics.

ACTIVE COSMETICS, OR COSMECEUTICALS

Although the FDA does not recognize the term, "cosmeceutical" is widely used in the cosmetic industry to refer to those products that are marketed as cosmetics and that contain ingredients that deliver clinically measurable benefits to the appearance of the skin. Since they are not considered drugs, they are not regulated by the FDA. For example, antioxidants, polyphenols, alpha hydroxy acids, and retinol fall in this category.

In the chapters that follow, we highlight the most common skincare concerns, including acne and rosacea, skin discolorations, sensitive skin, lines and wrinkles, and bumps and growths. Information is provided about the causes of each, details on how to identify a particular condition, tips on lifestyle changes you can make, recommendations for tailoring your skincare regimen to meet your needs, and advice on when to visit a dermatologist.

So, raise your expectations and take control of the opportunity to leverage your newfound knowledge for the betterment of your skin. You'll soon be on your way to revealing the great skin you've always wanted.

⊃ Put Your Products to the Test

Before changing your skincare routine, ask yourself the following questions. Challenge yourself to answer these questions honestly with high expectations for results.

1. Are my products specifically labeled for my major skincare concern?

_____ Yes _____ No

2. Are they working for me?

_____ Yes _____ No

3. Does my product include a "drug facts box" on the back label or outer carton indicating an active ingredient?

_____ Yes _____ No

4. What results do I want to see from my skincare products?

_____

_____

_____

5. How committed am I to achieving the results I want?

_____

_____

_____

If you answered "No" to questions 1, 2, or 3, it is time for you to revisit your skin needs. Use the mirror activity from Chapter One to help focus your skincare goals and find the right treatment for you. Your skin deserves it!

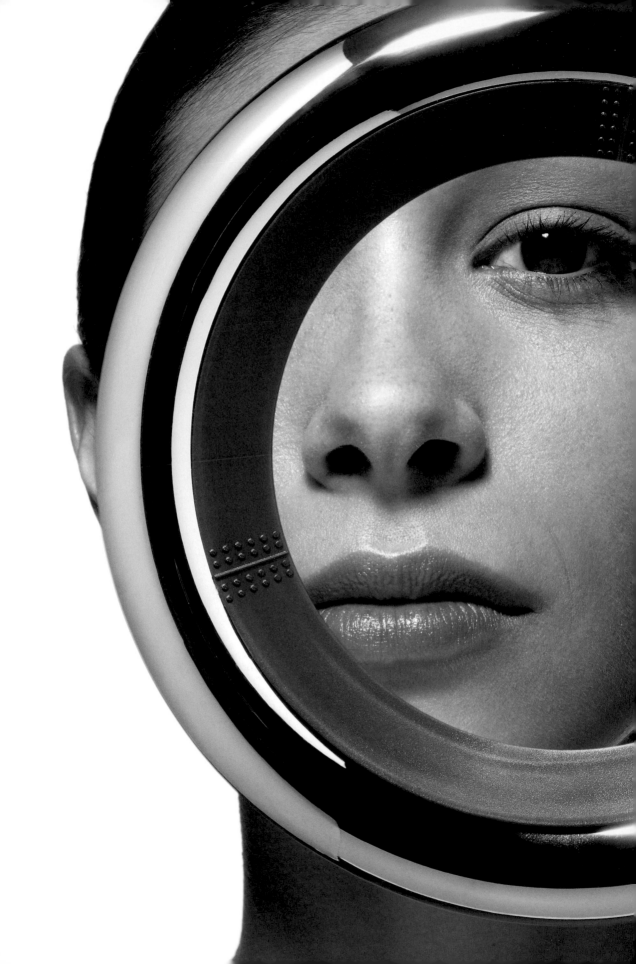

VISITING A DERMATOLOGIST

How to Feel the Love

"My visit to the dermatologist felt like 'drive-through medicine.' Pull up, present the affected body part, get a prescription, and leave. At least I got the Happy Meal prize: some free sunscreen samples."

Anonymous

W hat could be more demoralizing than sitting patiently in a doctor's waiting room, only to feel rushed or, worse yet, dismissed once you actually have facetime with your doctor? The unfortunate reality for us physicians is that our health care insurance system is under constant and very real cost pressure, and those pressures are transferred to the practitioner. With tightening reimbursement caps and specific price schedules assigned to medical diagnoses, many of our dermatology colleagues find that the only way to cover soaring overhead costs is through taking on more and more patients. Some of us are seeing up to forty patients a day. That's one every six minutes, and this trend doesn't show signs of slowing.

When Doctors Become "Health Care Providers"

As most of the country's ten thousand dermatologists are concentrated in major metropolitan areas, our ability to serve the skin, hair, and nail needs of three hundred million Americans is continuously challenged. Worse yet, with so few dermatologists seeing so many patients, procuring an appointment, especially with a popular doctor, may be an exercise in frustration or even rejection.

It is the plight of those seeking medically guided skincare advice that led us to write this book to empower you to self-treat common skincare concerns whenever possible. However, if you are not totally satisfied with your self-treatment and a trip to the dermatologist is warranted, this chapter will help ensure this visit will be a successful, even enjoyable, one.

How to Make Your "Derm Connection"

When it comes time to seek professional care for a medical or cosmetic concern, you should first determine whether it is a dermatologist you really need to see. For some concerns, especially related to foot conditions such as corns, calluses, and, on occasion, athlete's foot, a podiatrist might be a more accessible alternative. Also, if changes in skin are the result of other underlying health conditions, another medical specialist might better support your treatment plan. That's why some health insurance plans require a referral to a dermatologist, whether it is for acne, psoriasis, or even full-body mole checks. However, when a "gatekeeper" physician keeps you from accessing a dermatologist, it may be worth challenging. For instance, only board-certified dermatologists are, under FDA regulation, able to prescribe Accutane. In cases of severe acne, this most aggressive form of treatment can have profound benefits, not only for clearing skin but also in the resultant outcomes of self-esteem and even mental health.

Generally, dermatology visits for medical purposes are covered by health insurance plans. However, plans differ, so your first step should be to consult with your insurance provider to receive a list of board-certified dermatologists in your region who are covered by your plan. And before you make your appointment, double-check with your insurance company to make sure your particular issue is in fact covered. If you have the luxury of going outside your plan or if you are seeking a cosmetic dermatologist for treatments that are not covered by insurance, ask trusted friends, search the American Academy of Dermatology database at www.aad.org, or ask your general physician for a recommendation.

When selecting a cosmetic dermatologist, it is valuable to get a referral from someone who has achieved results you find attractive and who can provide you with specific insights about the appointment and the doctor's approach. Keep in mind that there is a real artistry in cosmetic dermatology. You may find a board-certified dermatologist with top training and education, but that doesn't necessarily mean he or she has an aesthetic eye. We urge you to do your homework when looking for this kind of specialist. Remember that many wealthy celebrities receive regrettable treatments, so don't just assume the most expensive dermatologist in your area can offer the best treatments.

Another important quality in selecting a doctor is finding someone thorough and committed to follow-up. You want to find a doctor who recognizes when problems arise, returns calls, and works with you through the entire condition, from treatment to resolution.

So you find the perfect dermatologist for you and then, gasp, he or she is not accepting new patients. What do you do? Ask for a referral! Most doctors will be happy to refer you to another well-qualified dermatologist. Although this is a great place to start, you'll still want to research this new dermatologist to make sure he or she meets your criteria.

When Should I See a Dermatologist?

We recommend that everyone see a dermatologist for a baseline full-body skin check at the age of twenty-five and every six to twelve months thereafter if there is a family or personal history of skin cancer. This visit is generally covered by insurance.

Is a Dermatologist Really a Doctor?

You may remember the following bit from a *Seinfeld* episode a few years back:

Jerry: [She] just spent an hour and a half making me feel if I don't save lives, I'm worthless.

Elaine: Well, she's very focused. Dermatology is her life.

Jerry: Dermatology?

Elaine: Yes, she's a dermatologist.

Jerry: Saving lives? The whole profession is: eh, just put some aloe on it.

George: Saving lives? She's one step away from working at the Clinique counter!

Jerry: Dermatologist? Skin doesn't need a doctor!

George: Of course not! Wash it, dry it, move on!

Just to clear up any confusion about the medical expertise, dermatologists are, in fact, physicians who specialize in the diagnosis and treatment of skin diseases from rosacea to melanoma. We have completed medical school, residency, and passed medical board exams.

Dermatology Subspecialties:

Dermatologic surgeons practice skin cancer surgery, including Mohs micrographic surgery, which is generally used to remove skin cancers on the face.

Immunodermatologists specialize in the management of skin diseases caused by compromised immune systems including lupus, AIDS, dermatomyositis, scleroderma, and Raynaud's disease.

Pediatric dermatologists specialize in the diagnosis and treatment of genetic and acquired skin diseases of children.

Cosmetic dermatologists focus on surgical and nonsurgical aesthetic procedures for the skin, including skin resurfacing, laser, and dermatological fillers, many of which we describe in Chapter Sixteen.

For other skin concerns, make an appointment on an "as needed" basis. For instance, make an appointment if you have unsightly skin growths or a mole that is changing in size, shape, and color. Don't feel reluctant or embarrassed to make an appointment because you feel that common conditions such as acne are simply "part of life." Most issues are treatable, so you shouldn't continue to live with or worry about them. And keep in mind that if you find a growth you are concerned about and cannot get an appointment with a particular physician, seek another dermatologist immediately. Because there is the potential that the scary-looking spot is a melanoma, time is of the essence.

Preparing for an Office Visit

We know that visiting any type of doctor can be intimidating. The following tips should help you prepare for your dermatology visit so you leave the office feeling satisfied that your needs have been met.

- *Come to your appointment with a list of questions you have prepared beforehand. Make sure you prioritize them in order of importance because the reality is that your doctor will have limited time to spend with you and additional follow-up visits may be required to address them all. Don't be insulted if your doctor will not answer cosmetic questions during a visit scheduled for medical purposes. He or she likely scheduled only enough time to deal with your primary concern.*

- *A day or two before you see your dermatologist, scan your entire body for potential skin, hair, and nail issues. Note anything that warrants discussion. This might include plantar warts, dry, itchy skin, "broken" capillaries, or toenail fungus, just to name a few.*

- *Since full-body skin checks are not always routine, if that is your request, let the scheduler know ahead of time to allow ample time during your appointment. When you meet with your doctor, you should point out all the moles that may have changed or appeared since your last visit.*

- *Be a proactive patient, particularly when it comes to negotiating with your insurance provider. Negotiating reimbursement prior to your medical visit can help you avoid unexpected out-of-pocket costs.*

- *Finally, manage your expectations (not all the services you may want will be covered by insurance, your doctor may not be able to address all issues in one visit, etc.) for a more satisfying experience.*

"I have patients who come in with pen marks circling the moles they want to have checked so they don't forget where they are. It's a simple trick that works very well for them and for me."

DR. KATHY FIELDS

A Typical Day at Our Offices

Heading to the dermatologist, especially for a cosmetic consultation, should be a relatively relaxing and enjoyable experience. We want to share some details about our own offices because it may give you a better sense of what a typical office visit can and should be like. Remember that you should be treated as a client by your dermatologist and his or her staff. Especially in a cosmetic practice, you are not just a patient; you are a livelihood.

Prescription for a Picture-Perfect Wedding?

A recent survey found that a major concern for brides as their big day approaches is a wedding breakout.[1] No woman should have to walk down the aisle with a zit on her cheek. What's the antidote? Relax! Stress releases the hormone cortisol, and increased levels of cortisol can increase the likelihood of a breakout. To help you stay calm, we recommend our patients schedule an appointment for the week of their wedding. Knowing they can see us if they need us for an "emergency zit fix" helps alleviate their worry.

Information to Bring to Your Dermatologist

You may think that doctors find it annoying when a patient comes in with a whole list of information and questions, but in reality, we love it because we can tailor the appointment to your needs. So be prepared. Here is some information you should share:

- Your dermatological history, including previous records (either bring your relevant records or have them sent ahead of time, and remember that doctors can't request records—only you can)
- Your main dermatological concerns in order of priority
- How long you have had a current condition
- What treatments you have tried to treat the condition; describe your results
- Medications you are taking, including over-the-counter analgesics such as aspirin
- Supplements and vitamins you are taking
- Any underlying illnesses you may have
- Skincare products you like or dislike or have sensitivities to

Our offices are staffed with enthusiastic, professional women who love what they are doing. They are approachable, encouraging, and will helpfully guide you through your initial questions. They have also tried many of the procedures we offer, so they can share thorough details and personal experiences when you set up your appointment.

As cosmetic dermatologists, our offices are filled with a lot of natural light so we can see your skin in the most revealing way. We start our appointments by handing you a mirror and asking you to show us what bothers you about your skin. We ask, "If you had a magic wand and could reduce, minimize, or eliminate something, what would it be?"

We have many options for treatment, so we want to get the best understanding of your expectations and desired final results. We often set up the first appointment as a consultation. We share information on the appropriate procedures for your concern, including downtime, costs, and expected final results. We have equipped our offices with the best technological devices available, which makes our work personally rewarding because the results can be so exceptional. We are on the cutting edge of technology and offer our patients the most current treatments available.

We will photograph you before treatment and then at follow-up appointments; this will help you see the real benefits, because most of the best results are natural and subtle. If you are receiving a potentially painful procedure, we will go out of our way to make you comfortable. We also provide cover-up makeup before you leave and set you up with the appropriate topical treatments to use at home to optimally care for your skin and protect the good work we've just done.

"Patients often go through their list of questions and then say 'Oh, by the way....' It turns out that question is usually what they should have brought to my attention first. Remember that the subject that seems most embarrassing is probably the most urgent. Don't be shy; it is really important for your health and well-being to tell us what is going on."

DR. KATIE RODAN

And remember that we like follow-up from your end as well. If you feel our staff treated you especially well and you are delighted with your results, let us know. We chose dermatology as our medical specialty because we personally know how empowering it is to feel good about your skin, so your satisfaction is our primary goal. A note to our staff about a positive experience means more than you know.

•

> Do Your Homework

Selecting the right doctor is never easy, be it for a general checkup, diagnosis on a mole, or laser treatment. Use this quiz to see whether you are on the right track.

1. Are you seeing a dermatologist for:
_____ A. Skin cancer
_____ B. Skin disease caused by immune system problems such as lupus, AIDS, or dermatomyosits
_____ C. A pediatric concern
_____ D. Aesthetic procedures such as skin resurfacing, lasers, and dermatological fillers
_____ E. None of the above

2. Is this dermatologist board certified by the American Academy of Dermatology?
_____ A. Yes
_____ B. No

3. Was this dermatologist referred to you by someone you know and trust?
_____ A. Yes
_____ B. No

4. How often does this dermatologist perform procedures such as lasers and fillers?
(Answer this question only if you picked "D" for question 1.)
_____ A. Frequently (every day)
_____ B. Occasionally (one to two times per week)
_____ C. Rarely (less than once per month)

Scoring:

Question 1:
A = see a dermatologic surgeon
B = see an immunodermatologist
C = see a pediatric dermatologist
D = see a cosmetic dermatologist
E = see a general dermatologist

Question 2:
A = +5/B = -10

Question 3:
If you answered "D" to question 1, A = +3/B = -4
If you answered "A," "B," "C," or "E" to question 1, A = +1/B = 0

Question 4:
If you answered "D" to question 1, A = +4/B – +2/C = -2
If you answered "A," "B," "C," or "E" to question 1, 0

Dermatologist's Score

6 to 12 points: Great work; you did your homework. This dermatologist has all the right qualifications. You should still analyze this doctor's qualifications, personality, office mannerisms, etc. Not everyone will be a great fit for you. You can also look online for reviews from other patients. If you still feel good about this dermatologist, book an appointment today.

-7 to -3 points: Think again. Put good reviews aside. If this dermatologist is not board certified by the American Academy of Dermatology, you should continue your search. You deserve the best!

-14 to -6 points: Do your homework. Nothing comes easy. Spend some time researching dermatologists in your area, talk to friends and coworkers, and search reputable sites online. The first doctor you find isn't always the best option. Make sure to find someone who is board certified by the American Academy of Dermatology. Once you match those criteria, you can look for referrals and good online reviews.

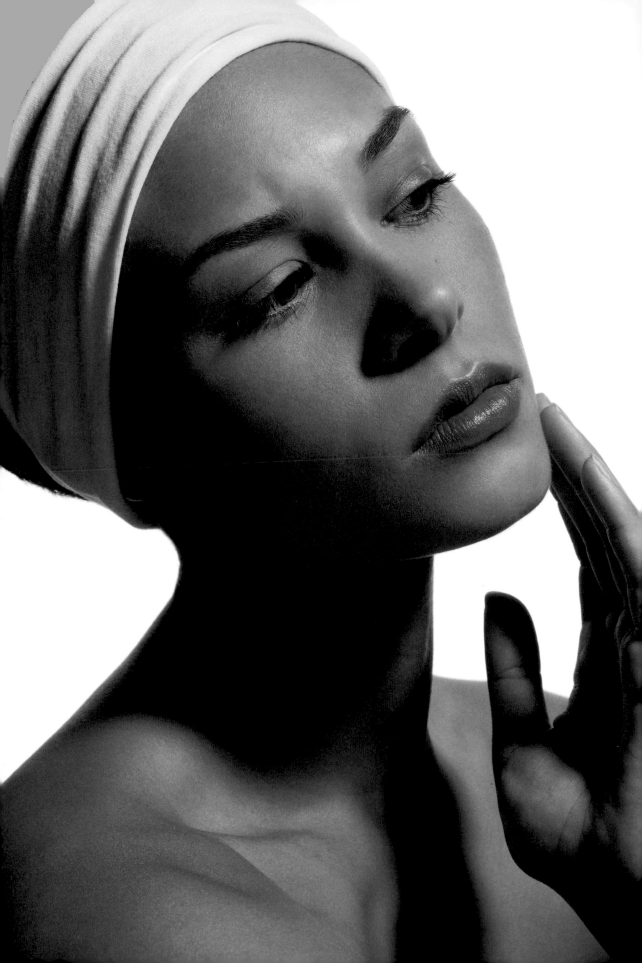

ACNE AND ROSACEA

They Impact Your Skin at Every Age

"The only good thing I can say about adult acne and rosacea is that if your face is red and bumpy, nobody will notice your wrinkles. When it comes to common skin concerns, breakouts trump everything."

Dr. Kathy Fields

You may have been plagued with pimples in high school and are watching history repeat itself through your teenage son or daughter. Or perhaps now, as an adult, you are experiencing breakouts for the first time. No matter what your age, skin type, or skin color, at some point, since you're human after all, you are bound to get a pimple. No one is immune. In fact, the American Academy of Dermatology reports that nearly 85% of people experience acne at some point in their lives.[1] It's not surprising that acne is the most frequently diagnosed condition at dermatologists' offices and the most common skin disease that exists today. But take heart: we've made it our mission to help all acne sufferers take control so that the physical and emotional challenges of this ubiquitous skin condition no longer need be a fact of life.

What Is Acne?

So you think you just get breakouts but don't have acne? Think again. Whether it's occasional breakouts associated with your monthly menstrual cycles, blackheads on your nose and chin, a full Class IV case of teenage acne, or embarrassing pimples on your back, chest, or even more unspeakable places, it's all acne in one form or another. Because a comprehensive plan of attack to clear your skin involves interrupting the processes that create the visible acne breakouts, we believe it behooves us to "put on our lab coats" and provide you with a basic understanding of how acne happens.

Acne vulgaris, the technical medical term, includes everything from a few blackheads, whiteheads, and inflamed pimples to deeper, more painful cysts and nodules. Acne is an inflammatory condition of the skin that occurs inside a pore—the passageway from the bottom of the hair follicle to the skin's surface. The bump that appears on your face is actually the final step in a silent process that begins deep inside a pore one to two weeks before the pimple is ever visible. Here's a simplified look at how acne forms:

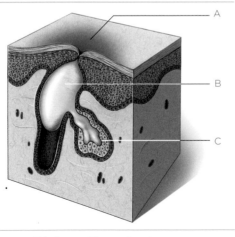

Skin layer with acne forming
A: Inflammation
B: Dead skin cells, sebum (oil), and bacteria
C: Sebaceous (oil) gland

STEP 1: CLOGGED PORES

During the normal process of skin renewal, skin cells that line pores are continuously sloughed, making room for fresh, new cells. But sloughing doesn't always happen as it should. Sometimes dead skin cells combine with skin's natural oil and instead of shedding, they clump together inside of a pore. A hard, firm plug called a comedo is then formed inside the pore (think of it as a cork in a bottle), and the stage is set for acne to begin.

STEP 2: TRAPPING OF OIL (SEBUM)

Your hormones stimulate oil production in the sebaceous glands, which are attached to the pores. The plug (comedo) impedes the oil from traveling up through the pore to the surface of the skin, as it is meant to do. Instead, this oil is trapped and provides the ideal environment for bacteria to flourish. Keep in mind that this can happen even if you have dry skin.

STEP 3: BACTERIAL ATTACK

Once your pores are clogged, an airtight environment is created and anaerobic (oxygen-hating) bacteria called *Propionibacterium acnes* (*P. acnes* for short) "feeds and breeds" on the abundant oil, releasing inflammatory toxins. (Interesting fact: although the *P. acnes* bacteria must be present for acne breakouts to occur, there is not a clear correlation between the amount of *P. acnes* on the skin and the tendency to break out.)

STEP 4: INFLAMMATION

The body's response to these toxins is a swarming army of red and white blood cells sent to contain the infection. The end result is intense swelling, inflammation, and pain in the form of a pimple, pustule, or, in more severe cases, a cyst or nodule.

Additionally, some people continue to suffer the aftermath of acne in the form of a pink/brown discoloration (post-inflammatory hyperpigmentation) at the site of the healed blemish that lasts long after the acne has cleared. The darker your skin color, the more likely you are to experience these marks. Although many people confuse these with actual scars (see sidebar on next page), they are not permanent. However, they can be quite persistent and without treatment may take months or even years to fade. Like the acne itself, these marks can be treated, but preventing acne breakouts in the first place is a double win and is always your best bet.

The Emotional Impact of Acne

The emotional impact of acne can be significant. Kendra, seventeen, says, "I don't go to parties or talk in class because I don't want anyone to notice me. I don't even look in the mirror because I don't want to see myself. I hate the way I look and feel every single day."

Although far too many of us can relate to Kendra, our intention isn't to take you on a walk down a not-so-pleasant memory lane but to emphasize that the psychological damage of acne is real and significant. Several studies have shown that when people have acne, they also experience low self-esteem, social withdrawal, and depression, and some carry this negative emotional baggage with them throughout their lives. Cindy, a forty-five-year-old patient of Dr. Rodan's, confided that she felt she never lived up to her potential as an adult because of the acne she had as a teen.

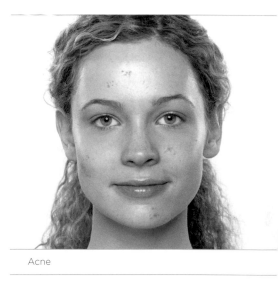

Acne

Although we are not psychiatrists, we witness such anguish daily. But unlike years ago when acne was a condition you just had to live with, today it can be treated fairly easily and quite successfully. This means no one, including Kendra and Cindy, has to live with the pain, anger, and depression of acne any longer.

If you're the parent of a teen with acne, it's important to open up the lines of communication and let your child know you're there as a support system. We sometimes encounter reluctance on the part of parents to treat acne when they first see it. Some don't realize it is quite treatable, and others seem to underestimate the role it plays in their child's life. Even mild acne can contribute to low self-esteem, self-consciousness, and poor body image. Helping a teen treat acne as soon as it begins can prevent more severe acne, reduce the risk of acne scarring, and, perhaps most important, deter lifelong stress.

True Acne Scarring

What is an acne scar?
A true acne scar (not to be confused with post-inflammatory hyperpigmentation), like all scars, occurs as a natural part of the body's wound-healing process and becomes a permanent reminder of injury and tissue repair. In terms of acne, scarring can take the form of depressed pits, broad indentations, or raised, thickened, round, or linear bumps called keloids.

Who gets acne scars?
Generally speaking, the more advanced cases of cystic and nodular acne are the most likely to cause scarring, so it is especially critical to take all possible measures to manage this condition. However, as with acne itself, some people are simply more likely to scar, especially those with a family history. If you have a parent who suffered from acne scarring, you may be at a greater risk of scarring as well. Predicting who will scar, however, is often quite difficult. "Severe" inflammation in some people may not result in scarring, while in others, a small pimple may leave permanent damage. And if you're inclined to pick, consider this: you're creating a wound on your skin, and nature is going to do what it must to quickly repair it, even if it's not pretty. So as tempting as it might be to teach that pimple a lesson by squeezing and picking, refrain and follow our advice for the emergency pimple fix later in this chapter.

How do you treat acne scars?
Unfortunately, we have an adage: "Once a scar, always a scar." There is no universally effective treatment to remove scars. However, you may be able to lessen the appearance with injections of fillers, laser treatment such as Fraxel, or even scar revision surgery. With this in mind, it's important to remember that prevention is key. Stop the acne and you'll stop the scars before they've had a chance to form.

Adults and Acne

If there's one thing we know about acne, it's anything but predictable. Therefore, our skin isn't necessarily out of the woods even after the trauma of puberty is behind us. In fact, approximately 30%–40% of women develop acne at one time or another during their adult years, with some suffering with it for up to twenty years. Like all acne, adult acne is triggered by a complex combination of factors, primarily genetics (your inherited predisposition to acne), hormones, environment, climate, stress, and medications. (For more on stress and acne, see Chapter Three.)

The difference is that as we age, pimples tend to move south on the face, with adults more commonly experiencing acne around the mouth and on the jawline, while teen acne tends to cluster on the forehead and cheeks. Overall, pimples on adults are fewer in number but bigger in size.

Am I Causing My Acne? Acne Myths and Astute Observations

MYTH: "My daughter doesn't wash her face enough, so she's breaking out."
FACT: Actually, maybe she's washing her face too much and causing oil rebound.

MYTH: "I've been on the phone all day, so I'm getting acne along my jawline."
FACT: Constant pressure and perspiration on an area may indeed contribute to irritation that leads to inflammation inside of your pores and ultimately to breakouts.

MYTH: "My friend eats a lot of greasy food; that's why she has pimples."
FACT: There is no proven correlation between dietary fats and breakouts.

In our patients' efforts to find an identifiable reason for acne, we repeatedly hear many misconceptions as well as some astute observations. Ironically, the stress of trying to figure it all out may be as relevant as any lifestyle factor that contributes to acne. Nonetheless, many myths have

Can Food Cause Acne?

The role of diet and acne remains controversial. Although the current dominant view among dermatologists is that food does not cause acne, several recent studies have pointed to some possible exceptions, namely, high glycemic diets and milk.

Loren Cordain, PHD, studied the eating habits of tribes in Paraguay and Papua New Guinea, where hunting, fishing, and gathering fruits and vegetables are the primary sources of nutrition. In these non-Western societies he found a complete absence of acne vulgaris in the populations (more than 1,300 people total). His hypothesis is that a traditional Western diet, high in refined carbohydrates, permanently boosts insulin. This in turn elevates growth hormone levels, stimulating the sebaceous secretions that lead to clogged pores and acne.[2]

A recent Australian study published in the *American Journal of Clinical Nutrition* supports the high glycemic diet/acne connection.[3] The study followed two groups of males ages fifteen to twenty-five. The first group continued to eat a diet high in sugar and processed grains, foods that have a high glycemic index. The other ate a diet high in whole grains, lean meat, and fish, fruits, and vegetables. After twelve weeks, the men in the group eating the low glycemic diet had 51% fewer pimples than when they started.

Another study conducted by a team of scientists at Harvard and published in the *Journal of the American Academy of Dermatology* examined the diets of 50,000 people. They found that people who consumed diets high in milk had more acne. They therefore concluded that an association exists between milk consumption and acne, hypothesizing that dairy products expose us to hormones that can lead to increased acne.[4]

developed around acne, and we thought this would be a good opportunity to debunk some of the most common.

MYTH: Acne is caused by poor hygiene.
FACT: Acne is caused primarily by internal, not external, triggers.

MYTH: Chocolate, pizza, and French fries cause acne.
FACT: The overall correlation between diet and acne is still unclear, so it's best to use common sense. If certain foods consistently seem to make you break out, you should avoid them. For example, some people are supersensitive to foods with a high iodine content such as shellfish, dried fish, and seaweed. Importantly, eating healthy will always serve you well and help your body resist the effects of inflammation and stress. As we like to say, "What's eating you may be more important than what you're eating." (See sidebar above for more information on acne and food.)

MYTH: I'm doing something wrong to cause my acne.
FACT: Acne is caused because of your genetics and hormones—it's not your fault.

MYTH: There is nothing you can do about acne. It is a "rite of passage" that everyone has to go through.
FACT: From topical treatments to medications, acne is very treatable. People no longer need to live with acne.

"When I was a teen, someone told me that brewer's yeast was good for acne because of the vitamin B in it. For the sake of clear skin, I drank a scoop of it in water every day, but it tasted horrible and caused my skin to flush. After a few months, I realized it wasn't helping a bit. This illustrates the desperate means I was willing to take for the sake of clear skin."

DR. KATIE RODAN

MYTH: Sunlight clears acne.

FACT: Although getting a tan on your face may immediately mask some of the redness and inflammation associated with acne, chronic sun exposure actually damages skin and makes your breakouts more likely to leave remnant pigment marks. The risks associated with sun exposure and not protecting your acne-prone skin with sunscreen far outweigh any perceived benefits.

MYTH: If you attack the blemish you see, you will cure the problem.

FACT: It takes a full one to two weeks for a blemish to surface. The bump that appears on skin is actually the final step in the process, making spot treatments largely ineffective. Skin needs targeted medicines that penetrate to where the problem originates, stopping acne before it's visible on the skin's surface.

The most important message to take away from this chapter is that, for most of us, although acne is a fact of life, life is better when we deal with acne than when we ignore it. Even an occasional monthly breakout is still considered acne. Staying ahead of these breakouts takes a commitment to treating the underlying causes of acne every single day.

When It Comes to Acne, Become a "Control" Freak

We cannot stress enough that although acne is not curable, it is treatable and controllable. Today there are lots of options, from topical treatments to low-dose oral contraceptives, to treat, control, and prevent future acne breakouts. But keep in mind that there are no quick fixes — once you get your acne under control, it may take many years of ongoing preventative treatment to keep your breakouts from resurfacing. And spot treating acne makes as much sense as brushing only the tooth with the cavity while ignoring the rest of your mouth. For a long-term solution, you must treat your entire face to stop the process that is happening deep inside your skin's thousands of pores.

Below we outline the treatments to attack each of the factors that contribute to the formation of an acne breakout. In all cases, whether your treatment is under the care of a physician with prescription medicines or self-directed with OTC options, the basic principles of treatment are the same: unclog the pores, kill the bacteria, and calm the inflammation.

Unclogging Pores (and Keeping Them Unclogged)

To prevent dead cells from clogging pores, they must be kept from clumping together. Additionally, the plug that begins to develop when oils and cells mix together must be broken down or prevented altogether. This requires delivering the right ingredients deep into pores. Salicylic acid, alpha hydroxy acids, retinoids, and sulfur are ingredients capable of disrupting the plug-forming

⊕ Acne and Self-Image

In an American Academy of Dermatology (AAD) study of 502 teens with acne, more than one-third of teens fifteen to seventeen say that acne has made them feel self-conscious, and one out of eight teenagers said they avoided looking in the mirror because they were embarrassed.[5] In a separate study conducted by the British Acne Support Group, 39% of British teens with acne said they had avoided going to school because of their skin, and 66% said their acne made them depressed.[6]

Gap Shown between Teens and Parents Regarding Psychological Aspects of Acne

A survey of 504 teens with acne and 500 parents of these teens sponsored by Galderma Laboratories LP and reported in *Dermatology Times* showed that parents consistently don't understand the negative impact acne has on the lives of their children. Thirty-six percent of the teens said acne created problems with their self-image while only 15% of parents thought this to be true. Additionally, 68% of parents believed they were supportive and understanding regarding teen acne, while only 48% of teens agreed.[7]

union of cells and oil to keep pores clear. For ongoing management of oil production, some physicians will prescribe oral contraceptives such as Yaz or Yasmine or an androgen-blocking agent such as spironolactone to their female patients.* In extremely severe acne cases, dermatologists may prescribe Accutane, a synthetic vitamin A derivative. Accutane may be prescribed only by a board-certified dermatologist and is preferentially prescribed to male patients because of the very high risk of birth defects associated with its use in pregnancy.

Killing Bacteria

Benzoyl peroxide is our preferred antibacterial agent for long-term control of acne, while oral antibiotics or other topical antibiotics such as clindamycin may sometimes be prescribed by physicians for short-term use. However, one of the risks of many antibiotics is the potential for bacterial resistance to develop. In the case of acne, many of the antibiotics that are used not only run the risk of leading to resistance of the P. acnes bacteria but also foster the development of resistant strains of Staphylococcus aureas and other problematic bacteria. Benzoyl peroxide, on the other hand, has not resulted in a single known case of bacterial resistance in more than forty years on the market. We recommend using benzoyl peroxide at 2.5%, the lowest clinically effective concentration. Medical studies demonstrate that a 2.5% benzoyl peroxide product is equally as effective in removing the P. acnes bacteria as a 10% product, with less potential irritation.

Treating Inflammation

While unclogging the pores and killing bacteria will keep new bacteria from forming, the most immediate improvement in acne comes from treating the swelling or inflammation. This will help reduce redness as well. Ingredients such as sulfur or oral antibiotics (tetracycline) are commonly used for their anti-inflammatory benefits. For a quick emergency acne fix, you can see your dermatologist for a cortisone injection to get rid of that one nasty pimple. It can shrink a blemish within twenty-four hours.

> **?DID YOU KNOW?**
>
> BENZOYL PEROXIDE IS MORE EFFECTIVE THAN ANTIBIOTICS FOR ACNE TREATMENT. A 2004 STUDY FOUND THAT TOPICAL BENZOYL PEROXIDE WAS MORE EFFECTIVE THAN THE MOST COMMONLY PRESCRIBED ORAL MEDICINES, TETRACYCLINE OR MINOCYCLINE, IN TREATING ACNE. [8]

Finally, treating the effects of post-inflammatory hyperpigmentation finishes the job that your antiacne routine starts. By clearing remnant dark marks with a product containing proven skin lightening benefits, you can achieve a clear, healthy-looking, radiant complexion. Remember that sunscreen is a critical component in reducing dark marks (or preventing them in the first place) and for ensuring optimal results.

The Evolution of Acne Treatments

Okay, so we're going to blow our own horn a bit here: acne treatment options have changed dramatically in the past couple of decades, largely because of the introduction of Proactiv Solution in 1995. Prior to that there were really only three options to treating acne, and most people were not getting the treatment they needed. You could use the available over-the-counter spot treatments, but spot treatments don't control acne; they're too little too late. You could see a dermatologist who could prescribe antibiotics, Retin-A, or even Accutane, but these can be highly irritating, expensive, and fraught with side effects, not to mention that many people don't have ready access to a dermatologist. Or, like most people, you could do nothing and wait for the acne to clear on its own.

But because acne can last an average of six to seven years in a teen and up to twenty years in an adult woman, the physical and emotional scars associated with "letting acne run its course" can

* These ingredients are available by prescription only.

The One That Got Away: An Emergency Pimple Fix

Apply ice buffered by a napkin for ten to fifteen minutes to reduce redness and telltale swelling.

Cleanse and apply a treatment lotion containing sulfur, which can be purchased without a prescription. Sulfur helps to unplug pores and shrink swelling.

Follow with a product containing 1% hydrocortisone or benzoyl peroxide (both are available over the counter) to keep pores freer and cleaner.

Apply a thin layer of a medicated concealer.

If time permits, get a cortisone shot from your dermatologist. The results can be miraculous.

be difficult if not devastating. These treatment limitations caused a lot of frustration for acne sufferers, which we were hearing about from our acne patients early in our careers.

As dermatologists and as women, we knew there had to be a better way for more people to access effective acne treatment. We set out to create an effective acne therapy through a system that incorporates multiple OTC medications in the right formulations used in the right order to target each required step in interrupting the acne process—unplugging pores, killing bacteria, and reducing inflammation. The net result is clear skin through acne prevention.

We're proud that we have been recognized by our professional and industry peers as revolutionizing the OTC acne category. However, no industry award is more meaningful to us than the reward of being able to help millions of people find the simple solution to their acne and regain the self-esteem that comes with clear, healthy skin.

On the Horizon

We regularly have the opportunity to see developments in the treatment of acne and are optimistic that new options will continue to provide alternatives to control acne and keep skin clear. One exciting area of research involves the use of small chains of amino acids, or peptides, for antimicrobial and anti-inflammatory benefits in treating acne. Early promise has led to continuing development of both prescription and cosmeceutical options for acne or acne-prone skin.

New devices have also recently hit the market for acne treatment. We've seen encouraging results with LEDs (light-emitting diodes) that treat skin with specific wavelengths of blue light and red light. Currently, LED treatments are available by appointment in some dermatology clinics, but these can be quite expensive and require regular visits to the clinic. There are also home-use units hitting the market. People who use these units to treat a single blemish report that the blemish heals faster than when left untreated. Such light treatment may ultimately prove beneficial for isolated blemish care, but to truly keep acne in check, there is still no substitute for full-face daily medicated skincare.

Rosacea

Like acne, rosacea ("roh-ZAY-sha") has a major impact on sufferers' quality of life. Painfully visual, it is often a stigmatizing disorder because it has been inappropriately associated with heavy drinking thanks to the noticeable rosacea symptoms seen in known alcoholics such as WC Fields. And like acne, the psychological impact of the disease is often more severe than the condition itself.

In a recent survey of more than four hundred rosacea patients conducted by the National Rosacea Society, 76% said their condition had lowered their self-confidence and self-esteem, 70% had feelings of embarrassment, and 52% reported that rosacea had caused them to avoid public contact or cancel social engagements. Among rosacea patients with severe symptoms, nearly 70% said the disorder had adversely affected their professional interactions and nearly 30% said they had even missed work because of their condition.[9]

The fact is, more than seventeen million Americans suffer from rosacea (think Bill Clinton's ruddy complexion), a condition in which the blood vessels of the skin dilate and constrict easily in response to a variety of stimuli including spicy food, alcohol, embarrassment, heat, sunlight, and the hot flashes of menopause. Women are more than three times as likely as men to exhibit it, although the symptoms are often more pronounced and severe in men. While this is an extremely common skin disease, it is grossly misunderstood, often misdiagnosed, and frequently improperly treated.

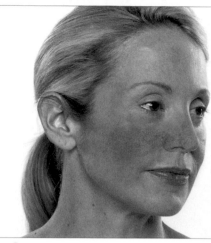

Rosacea

How Do I Know Whether I Have Rosacea?

Rosacea is characterized by intense and frequent flushing or blotchy redness, the appearance of "broken blood vessels" on the cheeks, chin, and nose, and in most cases, acnelike pimples. In fair-skinned people, particularly of Scottish, Irish, and English descent, early signs of rosacea may be the pink, flushed cheeks of youth. Eventually, rosacea progresses to a permanent redness of the midface, cheeks, nose, and chin, along with pustules and red inflammatory acne bumps. Rosacea is often incorrectly referred to as adult acne, but it lacks the comedones (blackheads and whiteheads) of acne vulgaris.

The exact causes of rosacea are unknown, but it is clear that it runs in families. If you suffer from rosacea, you probably also have some components of sensitive skin. Additionally, we believe hormones play a strong role, as many women notice rosacea flares when they are menstruating or during the menopausal years. There are also theories that suggest an infectious component such as *H. pylori* bacteria or *Demodex folliculorum*, a certain type of microscopic mite, may play a role. This mite, a normal resident in human skin, lives in hair follicles. Two recent studies revealed that the mites were significantly more numerous in facial skin samples of people with rosacea than in people without the condition. In addition, the mite population peaked on the skin samples of these patients in the spring, when rosacea tends to flare up.

We can sometimes identify pre-rosacea in teenagers and women in their early twenties. They may come to see us with concerns about acne, but because of the "flush and blush" syndrome, we know they are experiencing the early signs of rosacea. Like acne, rosacea is not curable, so we advise our patients to educate themselves, avoid the triggers, and treat the symptoms in an effort to minimize the intensity and frequency of flare-ups.

How to Treat Rosacea

Although rosacea cannot be cured, there are a variety of treatments available that can help keep it under control. The most common treatments include oral antibiotics, in particular within the tetracycline family, and topical antibiotics such as metronidazole. Topical agents such as azelaic acid, benzoyl peroxide (because *P. acnes* may also play a role in rosacea), sulfacetamide (10%), and sulfur (5%) are also often used as treatment. Advances in peptide technology have been found to be effective at calming inflammation associated with rosacea.[10]

Rosacea Triggers

- Sun exposure

- Red wine

- Smoking

- Heat—hot or steam baths, radiant heat, saunas, warm environments

- Spicy foods

- Hot drinks

- Caffeinated beverages

- Cosmetics and skincare products containing high levels of alcohol or acetone, as well as fragranced products

- Anxiety, embarrassment, and stress

- Physical exertion

Sometimes rosacea will flare up with the application of rich emollients, glycolic acids, or astringents containing alcohol. Therefore, rosacea sufferers must be extra cautious in their selection of skincare products. Cleanser selection is particularly important, and emulsion-type soap-free options are generally best. Look for physical sunblocks containing zinc oxide because physical blockers reflect the uv light back into the environment instead of absorbing it and turning it into heat energy, as chemical sunscreens can. These physical blocking agents also keep the skin cool and therefore less likely to flush.

Although there are no over-the-counter medicines approved for treating rosacea, choosing skincare products that are formulated for hyperirritable skin may help keep skin calm and less likely to react adversely. Products for sensitive skin with optical filters or a slight green tint can help to reduce the appearance of redness and ruddiness as well.

If the chronic effects of rosacea have left you with persistent redness, newer, highly effective methods for treatment consist of cutting-edge pulsed dye laser (PDL) and nonlaser intense pulsed light (IPL) therapies. The redness can be dramatically reduced after a series of five to six fifteen-minute treatments. However, you may need occasional maintenance treatments forever. The pulsed dye laser is better for reducing the appearance of thicker blood vessels, while intense pulsed light treatments are better for fine vessels. We will talk more about the details of these laser treatments in Chapter Sixteen.

A recent study by Tan and Tope and reported in the *Journal of the American Academy of Dermatology* looked at the effects of treating sixteen patients with signs of rosacea with PDL.[11] After just one treatment, every patient in the study experienced significant improvement. With two treatments, redness decreased by 40% to 60%. Patients also reported reductions in flushing, burning, itching, dryness, swelling, and sensitivity, which they said significantly improved their quality of life.

A discussion with your dermatologist will help you determine whether either therapy is right for you.

If Your Skin Has You Seeing Red...

When your skin is challenged with either acne or rosacea, getting your condition in check is your first skincare priority. Leaving acne and rosacea unchecked will cause changes in your skin that further accelerate the appearance of aging. Once you are in control of your acne or rosacea, you can strategically add the right kind of antiaging ingredients to your routine on a judicious basis.

> Is It Acne? Is It Rosacea?

1. Do you get blackheads?

_____ Yes   _____ No

2. Are your lesions distributed on your skin, forehead and/or t-zone?

_____ Yes   _____ No

3. Do you have pustules?

_____ Yes   _____ No

4. Are your lesions distributed evenly on your face but mostly concentrated on your midcheeks?

_____ Yes   _____ No

5. Do you easily flush/blush in response to alcohol, sun exposure, embarrassment, and heat exposure?

_____ Yes   _____ No

6. Do you have permanent facial redness, i.e., "broken capillaries"?

_____ Yes   _____ No

7. Do you have increased skin thickening and bumpiness of the nose, i.e., rhinophyma?

_____ Yes   _____ No

8. Do you have burning, irritation, or slight stinging of yours eyes, with a "blood shot" appearance?

_____ Yes   _____ No

9. Do you frequently have eyelid sties?

_____ Yes   _____ No

If you answered "Yes" to questions 1–2, you most likely have acne. If you answered "Yes" to questions 3–9, you may have rosacea. If you answered "Yes" to a combination of questions 1–9, you may have both acne and rosacea. Refer back to this chapter for appropriate treatment.

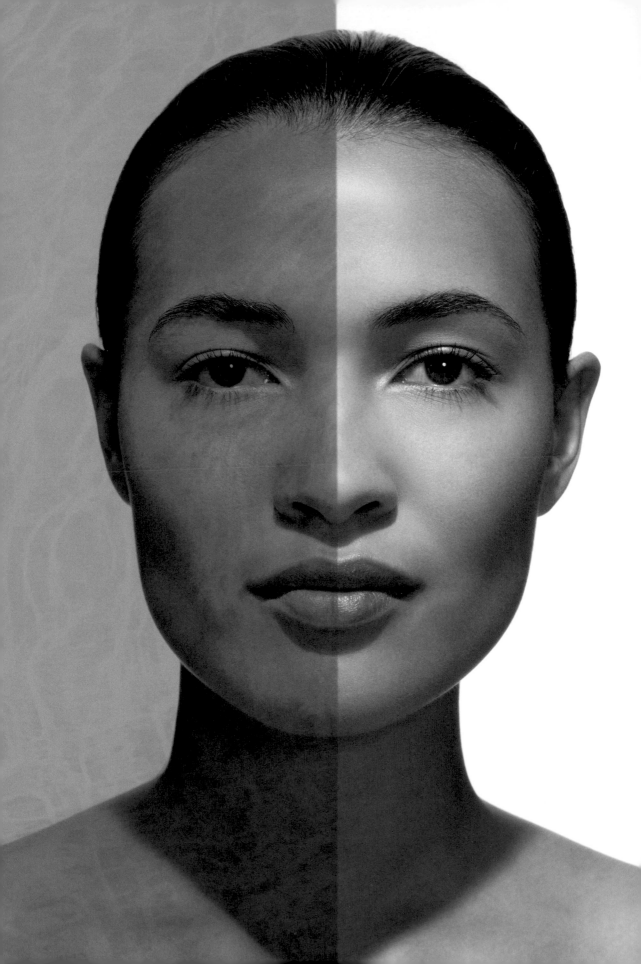

SKIN DISCOLORATIONS

They Impact Your Skin at Every Age

"I've done it all, Botox, lasers, fillers, you name it, but my skin still looks dull, drab, and spotty, like a muddy lake. Is there anything I can do to my skin to bring back the radiance and glow I see when I look at photos of myself when I was in my twenties?"

Linda, age forty-nine

When it comes to dull skin, it's generally not what you see that's the problem—it's what you don't see. Patients make appointments to see us for the obvious patches of unwanted pigmentation on the surface of their skin, but they'll rarely make an appointment for the problem they can't see—the changes beneath the surface that rob skin of its vibrancy. That's why we've spent countless hours demonstrating what happens as skin accumulates sun damage and how this is reflected in the mirror. Treating dull skin has become one of our most passionate crusades because once the problem is recognized, treatment is simple, and the results are typically amazing.

Now You See It…

We use a tool called uv reflectance photography to help see sun damage that is not visible to the naked eye. By taking a Polaroid picture using a uv flash, we can observe what is happening several millimeters beneath the surface of the skin.

When the skin's pigment melanin is evenly distributed through the cell layers of the epidermis, the light from the uv flash reflects evenly, resulting in a facial photo that appears consistent in tone.

On the other hand, the uv camera will highlight areas of abnormal and uneven melanin production, which appear as dark marks in the Polaroid. While not obvious to the naked eye, the presence of these subsurface discolorations explains why the skin appears dull and aged.

We like to use the analogy of a lake. If you look at a muddy lake with a lot of particulate matter, sunlight is absorbed and scattered rather than reflected off the surface, which makes the lake look murky and drab. When the lake is free of muddy particles, light is perfectly reflected throughout the water, giving it a clear and translucent appearance.

Similar to a muddy lake, excessive pigmentation below the skin's surface absorbs light and reflects dullness. When your skin is free of excessive subsurface pigmentation, your complexion looks younger, brighter, and more even toned.

Sun Damage: Play Today, Pay Tomorrow

Much of what is written off as part of the normal aging process is really evidence of sun damage, an accelerated form of aging. Just compare your face, which is constantly exposed to the sun, to a protected area such as your fanny—the texture, quality, and color are completely different. Although the sun's burning uvb rays play a role, it's the more insidious uva rays that are the real culprit. Your skin is exposed to these uva rays 365 days a year in all daylight hours, rain or shine, and even through glass windows.

Because uv rays are so damaging to your DNA, nature gave your skin a mechanism for protecting itself from uv radiation: skin's pigment, or melanin. But nature doesn't care whether that pigment is even or not. It just wants to protect your DNA so your cells continue to replicate normally. Thus, every time unprotected skin is exposed to uva rays, a signal is sent to your pigment-producing skin cells, or melanocytes, to produce more melanin. Over time, this repeated stimulation causes the abnormal clumping of pigment beneath the skin's surface in the areas that are most frequently exposed. You will often see evidence of this in your late twenties as dull, drab, uneven skin tone. If left untreated, these discolorations appear as liver spots or larger brown patches.

This evidence of sun damage is cumulative and doesn't simply appear overnight. You may look in the mirror and notice one small brown spot on your cheek or nose, and your immediate reaction may be to try and target that particular spot. However, attempting to lighten an individual discoloration doesn't address the larger issue that is looming under the surface and causing a lackluster complexion.

When we examine the photos taken with our UV cameras, we can tell a lot about your past, and we can predict your future. If during your childhood you wore big sunglasses or had bangs that covered your forehead, those protected areas will not show the same extent of damage. If you spend hours a day commuting, the left side of your face will eventually demonstrate greater evidence of sun damage compared with the right. Using a UV photograph also tells us what may lie ahead: increasing dullness and eventually mottled pigmentation or age spots on the surface of your skin.

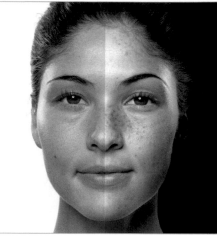

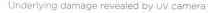
Underlying damage revealed by UV camera

Hyperpigmentation: The Pigment Changes You Can See

When it comes to aging, you might be focused on that wrinkle, but hyperpigmentation may have more of an impact than you think. In 2006, the *Journal of Evolution and Human Behavior* reported a breakthrough study that demonstrated the impressive impact skin pigmentation patterns have on the perception of age.[1] Digital photos of a woman's face were overlaid with different pigmentation patterns: that of a twelve-year-old, a forty-two-year-old, and a fifty-five-year-old. Four hundred thirty study participants were then asked to estimate the age of the woman in the photos. The study showed as much as a twenty year span in estimates associated with nothing more than the distribution of pigment on the skin.

Pigment distribution on the skin changes throughout a lifetime for a number of reasons, but there are generally three sources for the loss of uniformity and the appearance of unwanted marks or dark patches on skin:

- *sun damage in the form of brown or age spots*

- *hormonal changes in combination with UV exposure and/or heat in the form of melasma*

- *inflammatory processes called post-inflammatory hyperpigmentation in the form of dark marks that follow healed acne or trauma to the skin*

What's the Difference between a Freckle and an Age Spot, Besides Age?

Freckles, sun spots, brown spots, or age spots are different manifestations of uneven pigment distribution. We all know what freckles look like: they're pale to dark small spots of pigment scattered over the face, shoulders, back, and/or chest, most often on fair-skinned individuals. They usually begin to appear in childhood,

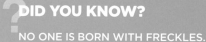
?DID YOU KNOW?
NO ONE IS BORN WITH FRECKLES.

but, contrary to what many will claim, nobody is born with freckles. While there is a genetic tendency to form freckles, exposure to sun is a critical factor in bringing them out. That is why freckles tend to be darker in the summer and may fade almost completely in the winter.

The same process that produces freckles in youth causes age spots, or solar lentigenes, with advancing age. These discrete dark spots prevalent on sun-exposed areas such as the face and the back of the hands and arms are simply larger versions of freckles.

The mystery remains, however, as to why these spots are so randomly and often distantly distributed. One theory is that the pigment-producing cells, melanocytes, have a tendency to migrate in the skin as we age. When two melanocytes find themselves in close proximity and are stimulated by uv light to produce excess pigment, there is a high possibility an age spot will form.

Solar lentigenes are found more often in fair-skinned individuals and are, in fact, present in 90% of Caucasian Americans older than sixty and 20% younger than thirty-five. Once discoloration is present, it is often permanent unless treated and will only get darker and more pronounced with continued sun exposure. Although "brown spots" are benign, they do indicate excessive sun exposure, which is a risk factor in the development of skin cancer.

Melasma

When increased circulating estrogen-type hormones are present in the skin of women, especially during pregnancy, patches of discoloration may appear along the outer margins of the face and above the upper lip. This condition, technically known as melasma, also occurs in women taking birth control pills or hormone replacement therapy and is known as the mask of pregnancy. It may come on quickly, sometimes appearing within hours of sun exposure. Although melasma may diminish after pregnancy, it often remains for many years or even a lifetime and may be very difficult to treat. But because the formation of discoloration is attributed to the reaction between increased circulating hormones in the body and the presence of uv radiation from the sun, prevention starts with diligent use of sun protection.

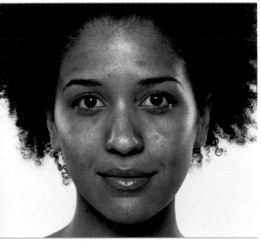

Post-inflammatory hyperpigmentation

Post-Inflammatory Hyperpigmentation (PIH)

Post-inflammatory hyperpigmentation (PIH) are those nasty souvenirs of a bad experience, be it acne, an allergic skin reaction, a bad trip to the waxing salon, or a cut or other skin wound. Although PIH is very common, particularly in darker skin tones, it is quite bothersome nonetheless. If the trauma has affected only the top epidermal layer of the skin, PIH can last for months or even years without medical treatment. But if the trauma is severe, affecting deeper dermal layers of the skin, the marks will be permanent, an unfortunate natural tattoo. PIH related to acne can be as upsetting as the breakout itself because while the pimple may have healed in two weeks, the post-acne brown spots may last for months.

To prevent PIH from occurring in the first place, shield any blemish or wound, no matter how small, from the sun (the sun makes dark spots darker). For minor injuries, be sure to apply a topical antibiotic such as Polysporin ointment and keep the area covered with an adhesive bandage to heal faster and without a scab. Contrary to popular belief, a scab is not a good thing when it comes to healing. Nature wants a wound to be protected. If you don't provide this protection, your body will do it for you in the form of a scab. A wound that is kept moist with an antibiotic ointment and then covered will heal much more beautifully than a wound that is allowed to take its natural course.

Treating Hyperpigmentation

Whether it's dullness associated with sun damage beneath the surface of your skin or obvious pigmented changes that are visible for all to see, you will be best served by treating the whole face. The approach is to exfoliate, lighten and brighten, and protect.

The regimen we are about to recommend has proven time and again to make a real difference in the complexions of those who adhere to it. Although it requires both patience and dedication of at least two to four months, it can make you feel much more confident and can help you look years younger. And even when your goal is to banish melasma or an age spot, you'll be best served by treating your full face to tackle the changes that lurk beneath the surface. Keep in mind that it is important to incorporate all the following steps, because as many of our patients have confirmed, best results come when you diligently follow these steps.

> "The real secret to long-term management of hyperpigmentation is strict, daily, year-round use of sunscreens and skin brightening treatments to fade the abnormal pigment."
>
> **DR. KATIE RODAN**

STEP ONE: EXFOLIATE

Removing dead skin cells helps to accomplish at least three important functions:

- *it accelerates turnover of the dead skin cells that contain excess melanin*

- *it clears the way for penetration of active treatment ingredients*

- *it refines skin's surface for more even light reflection and luminosity*

By using a cleanser that contains exfoliating properties, particularly those with gentle cleansing grains, alpha hydroxy acids, acetyl glucosamine, and retinol, it's easy to incorporate exfoliation into a skincare routine. Exfoliation offers a simple way to get your skin to act like it's younger

Types of Exfoliators

Chemical versus Mechanical Exfoliators

Not only are chemical and mechanical exfoliators quite different in composition but also their mechanism of action is different. Chemical exfoliators loosen dead cells by working between the layers of the epidermis, dissolving the links that enable the uppermost layer of cells to remain attached. This type of exfoliant can be found in facial cleansers, toners, moisturizers, and masks. The most popular chemical exfoliators are hydroxy acids such as glycolic acid, lactic acid, citric acid, and salicylic acid.

Mechanical exfoliators work by assisting in the physical removal of dead or excess cells. With either controlled abrasion or adhesion, mechanical exfoliators essentially polish the skin by immediately clearing the surface of dead, dulling cells. Cleansers and cleansing scrubs packed with sugars, salts, or polyethylene beads are our favorites. However, we recommend that you avoid harsh exfoliants that have sharp edges such as ground walnut shells and apricot pits. You also want to stay away from pads that feel like Brillo on your face. They can scratch the epidermis and leave skin raw, red, and reactive. Also be careful if you use body scrubs on your face—they tend to have larger particles and are made for stubborn areas such as heels and elbows, making them too aggressive for delicate facial skin.

We're fans of both gentle chemical and mechanical exfoliation, with the key word being "gentle." In our experience, it takes the perfect combination of the two to dissolve the bonds between cells without irritating skin and to sweep away dead cells, leaving skin soft and smooth. The secret is not to overdo it. If your skin looks red and angry after exfoliation, substitute a bland cleanser and moisturizer and give your skin a chance to recover.

than it is. Once you discover the right kind of exfoliation, your skin will look a million times brighter and healthier.

Procedures such as microdermabrasion and acid peels provide a deeper level of exfoliation. As long as they are not irritating to your skin, they may also enhance the skin's response to topical medication.

STEP TWO: LIGHTEN AND BRIGHTEN

To do this, we've found it's best to layer lightening and brightening agents, such as hydroquinone or vitamin C and retinol, onto the skin via varied delivery systems.

- *With a liquid vehicle, lighteners and brighteners quickly penetrate into the cells to interrupt the production of excess pigment. Using a toner that contains hydroquinone is an effective way to provide a rapid dose of this highly effective lightening agent to the skin.*

- *Following the above, apply a lotion or cream containing lighteners or brighteners, which provides a more sustained dose, for prolonged treatment.*

Other brightening ingredients include plant extracts such as bearberry or licorice, or ingredients such as kojic acid.

STEP THREE: PROTECT

Treating skin for hyperpigmentation without diligently protecting it from further UV exposure is like going up the down escalator. The UVA radiation will be triggering more pigment to be released as you are trying to slow it down. Thus, broad-spectrum sun protection containing zinc oxide, avobenzone, or Mexoryl is mandatory during the treatment process and forevermore if you want to keep the unwanted pigment from returning. In addition, wear protective clothing when in the sun. A single day of unprotected sun exposure can virtually undo months of treatment.

Skin Exfoliators

These ingredients help renew the skin by shedding surface cells that contain abnormal clumped pigmentation, allowing lightening agents or other active ingredients to more easily penetrate the skin. Be careful not to overdo exfoliation, which may cause inflammation and post-inflammatory hyperpigmentation.

- Alpha hydroxy acid

- Salicylic acid

- Peels (AHA/salicylic acids)*

- Microdermabrasion*

- Acetyl glucosamine

- Retinol

- Polyethylene beads

*procedures performed in a doctor's office

This simple skincare strategy should help restore the skin's clarity and brightness in the course of sixty to ninety days. However, many people tell us they see a positive change in their skin much sooner than that and their friends notice it as well. Once maximum lightening and evening of the skin have been achieved and the benefits have stabilized, you may want to change your routine to address another skincare issue.

Hydroquinone: The Gold Standard

Among dermatologists, hydroquinone is the mainstay in the treatment of unwanted pigmentation. It is the only FDA-recognized ingredient to lighten abnormal discoloration. It is available over the counter in 2% concentration and 4% by prescription. Although you can get the higher strength from your doctor, lower-concentration hydroquinone works extremely well when combined with exfoliation and sun protection. In addition, whereas prescription skin lighteners can be used only for a short period of time—usually not more than three months—lower concentrations can be used as long as it takes to get the job done without drying out or irritating the skin. In general, prescription-strength hydroquinone formulas are meant to be used only on those areas that require extra attention.

The benefits of a formulation containing hydroquinone for treating excess pigmentation can be boosted by botanical brighteners such as kojic acid, bearberry extract, arbutin, licorice, and salicylic acid, which help to even skin tone and reduce the appearance of dark marks and blotchiness. These skin brighteners are beneficial for brightening skin, but hydroquinone is the only OTC drug recognized by the FDA for skin lightening.

Patience and Commitment

Remember that your brown spots and discolorations took a lifetime to acquire, so a little patience in treating them will go a long way. While you may be tempted to jump right in, hydroquinone is a powerful medicine even at low doses. To get the best results, start a hydroquinone program slowly to allow your skin to accommodate.

Challenging the Gold Standard

While hydroquinone is our treatment of choice for lightening unwanted pigmentation, recent studies have shown that specific ratios of ascorbic acid (pure vitamin C) and retinol can yield impressive results.[2] This combination can be used continuously and offers added anti-aging benefits, such as improvement in lines and wrinkles. While we like these two ingredients, they don't like each other and cannot be stabilized in the same formula. To get the synergistic benefits of vitamin C and retinol, they need to be packaged separately and blended just prior to application. With this one-two punch, we believe the gold standard may have some competition.

In the first week, use medicated products every other day. In the second week, progress to once daily and by the third week twice daily as your skin begins to tolerate your new regimen. It is critical not to use hydroquinone on skin that is sunburned, windburned, dry, chapped or irritated or on an open wound.

The rationale for using a low concentration of hydroquinone over the entire face is to achieve a uniform complexion. Because hydroquinone works only on excessive pigmentation, it won't change your natural color. Nonetheless, spot treatments with prescription 4% hydroquinone often result in a halo affect, a white ring surrounding the brown mark.

The Big Guns

While we've continuously seen outstanding results with a simple OTC program for dull, unevenly pigmented skin, some discolorations are stubborn and resistant to this approach. In these more severe cases it is necessary to see a dermatologist for further options, including laser treatment. A doctor may also recommend a series of procedures such as microdermabrasion or acid peels to boost results from a topical lightening/brightening program by providing a deeper level of exfoliation and an enhanced uptake of the active ingredients. However, these procedures are not right for every skin type and run the risk of darkening pigmentation in some skin types. It is a good idea to work with your dermatologist to weigh the risks versus the benefits of these additional procedures.

Our Goal: Make the Need Obsolete

For achieving a dramatic improvement in the appearance of environmentally aged skin, we find that targeting pigmentation is the best place to start. Almost everyone sees compelling results within weeks. Once pigmentation is cleared and sun protection becomes a way of life, you can focus on other aspects of the aging face. In fact, with commitment to sun protection that includes sunscreens, protective clothing, and sun avoidance, the need for treatment of hyperpigmentation could conceivably become obsolete. Until that day, just remember: exfoliate, lighten, and protect.

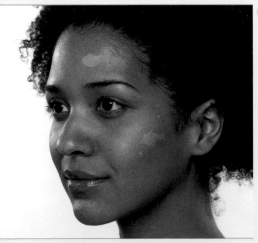

Vitiligo

What Is Vitiligo?

Vitiligo appears as large white patches on the skin that are devoid of pigmentation. It is an autoimmune condition affecting 1%–2% of the population and is most strikingly visible and disfiguring in people of color. Medical treatment includes topical steroids, tacrolimus, and the application of a photosensitizing agent followed by controlled UVA light exposure. Monobenzone or Benoquin is the treatment of last resort, permanently depigmenting any remaining unaffected areas to achieve an even color. Additionally, camouflage cosmetics can be helpful.

Sun Damage—Numbers Don't Lie!

Think you were born with those cute freckles? Think again. No one is born with freckles—they are all the result of sun damage, and we can prove it.

1. Count the number of freckles and moles on the inside of your right forearm.

_____

2. Count the number of freckles and moles on the outside of your left forearm.

_____

Notice a difference? The underside of your chin and your derriere, just like the inside of your forearms, are rarely exposed to the sun and are the best example of your true skin. Everything else is sun damage!

Want more conclusive evidence? Get a Wood's lamp (or black light), go into a pitch-black room, look into a mirror, and unveil your UV damage.

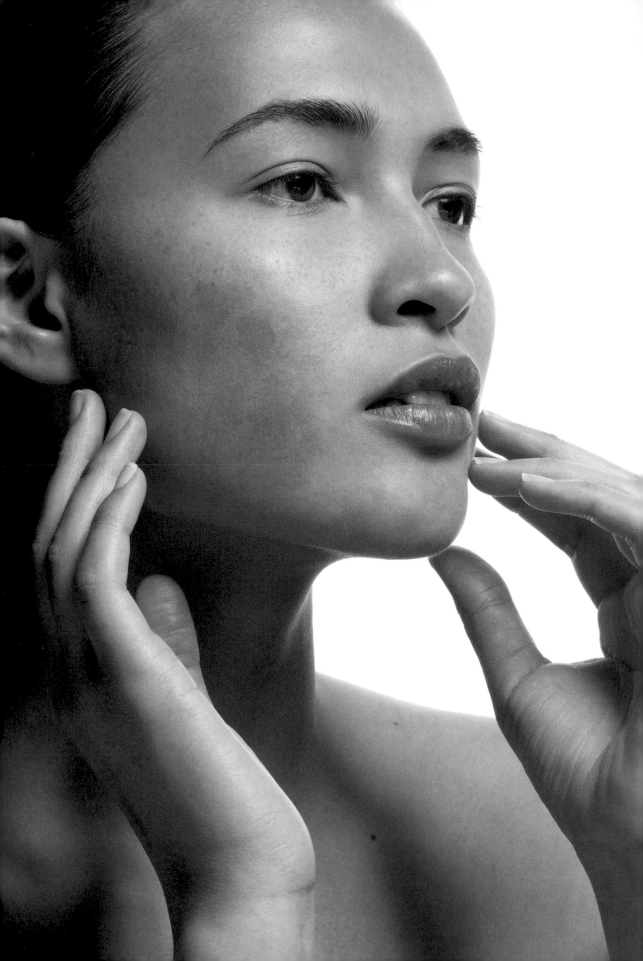

RED/SENSITIVE SKIN

"The eyes are the windows to the soul. But as dermatologists, we'll leave this romantic notion to the poets and philosophers and offer up for consideration a much more practical proposition: the skin is a reflection of the human condition."

Dr. Katie Rodan

T he appearance of your skin can speak volumes about what lies beneath. For instance, when the human body is stricken by infection, skin appears flushed due to fever. Gastric problems leave us looking pale, sometimes with a greenish tint. Cardiovascular disease may result in a bluish appearance to skin. Diabetic skin is at risk of ulcerated sores. Autoimmune conditions such as lupus can cause a butterfly rash on the face. Sensitive skin is telltale evidence of a reaction to an environmental irritant, allergen, or cosmetic product. It may produce dry, red, itchy patches in some people while in others cause a constellation of symptoms such as burning, stinging, tenderness, and itching without any visible changes.

Studies consistently tell us that more than 50% of women experience sensitive skin at some point in their lives. When tested, men show an incidence of skin sensitivity on par with women. Yet when surveyed, fewer men report their skin to be sensitive, hence the apparent rarity of "the sensitive male."

There are many reasons why the skin becomes sensitive. A small percentage of people have underlying skin conditions such as eczema or psoriasis, while a larger percentage are likely to have a genetic predisposition that makes them more susceptible to the impact of the environment, including stress, climate change, travel, sun exposure, cosmetic overuse, and mechanical irritation (friction or rubbing).

Genetic Predisposition, or Born to Need Mild

Within the first six months of life, approximately 20% of babies experience childhood eczema or atopic dermatitis—red, irritated, itchy skin that sometimes develops small, fluid-filled bumps. Just as asthma and hay fever allergies are evidence of an overreactive respiratory immune system, atopic dermatitis is evidence of an overreactive skin immune system. In fact, asthma and respiratory allergies often go hand-in-hand with eczema. Skin reactions are the by-product of hypervigilant immune system skin cells, called Langerhans cells, thrown into overdrive by stress or direct contact with environmental allergens. Even though childhood eczema generally clears by age twelve, the skin may be somewhat immunologically compromised and display evidence of sensitivity throughout life.

Other genetically influenced conditions that predispose us to sensitive skin, as a result of either the condition itself or its treatment, are seborrheic dermatitis, rosacea, or psoriasis. While all ethnicities are more or less equally prone to sensitive skin, the problem may manifest somewhat differently. For instance, rosacea is more prominent in those of us with fair complexions, and some studies report a greater incidence of sensory symptoms in Asian skin.

If you are genetically predisposed to sensitive skin, you will need ongoing management. Although there is no cure, it can be controlled very effectively in the short term through a combination of avoidance and treatment. Learn what triggers your reactions and decrease contact with soap and even water, as this makes skin dryer and more permeable. Talk to your doctor about medications such as antihistamines for the itch and cortisone for the more typical allergic reactions. First and foremost, you need to treat the underlying condition (described later in this chapter) and not just the symptoms.

Transient Sources of Sensitivity

A host of factors may affect skin sensitivity from time to time or even for long periods of time. And while many studies have been conducted to better understand whether and why some groups of people are more sensitive than others, there is much conflicting and inconclusive data.

Factors that may affect skin sensitivity include age (skin tends to become less sensitive as it ages), hormones, climate, and skin hydration, to name just a few. However, despite all the studies, the medical and scientific communities' ability to predict who will be sensitive to what is still

⊕ Will It Hurt?

Certain types of cosmeceutical ingredients will cause stinging among a percentage of the population. You can determine whether your skin is prone to stinging from specific ingredients in much the same way a skincare company would. First, expose your skin to a steam bath (a warm shower will do). Then apply the product in question to the nasolabial fold (the crease forming alongside your nose to the corner of your mouth) on one side of your face. To the other side, apply a mild product that you know your skin tolerates well. If you perceive stinging on the first side but not the other, you should proceed with caution as you incorporate the product into your skincare routine. You may still be able to use the product by starting slowly so that your skin can acclimate to the product over time. If persistent stinging, burning, or itching occurs, avoid the product altogether. Consider returning the product to the manufacturer and alerting it of your reaction.

not very good. The best we can do is to provide you with some tricks of the trade so that you and your skin can live harmoniously.

COSMETIC INTOLERANCE SYNDROME

In our experience, the vast majority of patients who suddenly exhibit sensitive skin without any prior history of it are really experiencing cosmetic intolerance syndrome. In other words, skin that's mad as hell and simply not going to take it anymore.

Read the labels. Between your personal care toiletries, skincare products, and makeup, you could be layering literally hundreds of chemicals onto your skin each day. You may realize that you've used too many strong products containing active ingredients and are experiencing product overload. There's even a possibility that ingredients in one product when combined with ingredients in another product are reacting together, causing your skin to experience heightened sensitivity.

Or perhaps you've been too aggressively exfoliating your skin, creating small, microscopic tears that predispose skin to moisture loss, infection, irritation, and less tolerance to other skincare products. If this is the case, you may find yourself experiencing the accompanying symptoms of burning, stinging, and redness.

STRESS AND YOUR SKIN

Stress can perturb the skin's protective barrier function, making you more likely to exhibit the signs of sensitive skin. As reported in a study in the January, 2001, issue of the *Archives of Dermatology*, when skin is stressed, it loses water at a greater rate, compromising its natural ability to continuously repair and renew itself.[1] Researchers examined the skin of twenty-seven students in three situations: just after returning from winter vacation (low stress), during final exams (high stress), and during spring break (low stress). They looked at how the skin responded to the repeated stripping of cellophane tape on the subjects' forearms during these various situations. They found it took longer for the skin to recover from the minimally invasive tape stripping during periods of perceived higher stress than during less stressful periods.

"Joan complained of burning and stinging when she applied anything to her skin, to the point of redness and rash. She brought in a suitcase full of the latest and greatest antiaging breakthroughs, which she was dutifully using morning and night, literally exposing her skin to hundreds of active cosmetic ingredients each day. As Joan's experience demonstrates, sensitive skin can be a manufactured and self-inflicted phenomenon among women. Some of us are simply overdoing it in an obsessive effort to be young."

DR. KATHY FIELDS

Another study conducted in 2007 by Theodore F. Robles, PHD, of the department of psychology at the University of California, Los Angeles, examined the effect of stress by dividing eighty-five participants into two task groups.[2] One group was assigned to a "no stress" (reading) task and the other to a "stress" (Trier Social Stress Test*) situation. Compared with the no stress condition, the stressed group showed delayed skin barrier recovery by 10% two hours after the tape-stripping skin disruption.

THE ENVIRONMENT

When you experience environmental changes such as traveling from a warm, moist locale to a dry climate with cold temperatures, low humidity, and wind, skin is much more likely to become sensitive. In the long term, chronic dryness may make the skin look more wrinkled and leathery, and prolonged scratching of the skin can produce lichenification—thick, dry, elephant-like skin.

When the barrier function is weakened through any of these means, the skin leaks moisture and its natural defenses can be compromised, allowing irritants, allergens, and infectious agents to more easily penetrate.

Psoriasis: Cells Gone Wild

WHAT IS IT?	TREATMENTS
Psoriasis is a common and chronic skin disorder that affects more than 7.5 million Americans, 25% of whom have a family history of it. The initial appearance of psoriasis can happen at any age. Once diagnosed, it is a lifelong condition. Generally people will experience dry, scaly patches of skin that are caused by a greatly accelerated rate of skin cell proliferation. These patches, called plaques, often appear on the elbows and the knees as well as the scalp and are generally not itchy. Those with psoriasis may go through bouts of remission, but then stress inevitably flares it up again. Environmental factors such as smoking, exposure to sun, and alcohol may affect how often psoriasis occurs and how long the flare-ups last.	Application of topical agents such as corticosteroids, vitamin D_3 derivatives, coal tar, or retinoids Light therapy administered in the physician's office (or a trip to the Dead Sea, the lowest point on earth, where the burning wavelengths [UVB] have been filtered by the atmosphere, leaving more UVA radiation, which has been shown to clear psoriasis) Oral medications such as retinoids, cyclosporine, and methotrexate and biologic agents such as Enbrel, Raptiva, and Humira that work on the immune cells may be used only after topical treatments and phototherapy have failed

*The TSST is a psychological procedure that allows experimenters to induce stress under laboratory conditions. It involves making a speech and performing an oral arithmetic task in front of an audience.

⊕ Ingredients That Are Good for Sensitive Skin

- Dimethicone
- Allantoin
- Oatmeal
- Chamomile
- Aloe vera

- Sulfur
- Lipids
- Vitamins C and E
- Green tea
- Dormins (plant bulb extracts)

What to Avoid

- Harsh mechanical exfoliants such as nutshells
- Chemical exfoliants such as salicylic acid and alpha hydroxy acids
- Propylene glycol
- Retinoids

- Alcohol
- Surfactants
- Fragrance
- Chemical sunblocks

Childhood Eczema: The Itch That Rashes

WHAT IS IT?	TREATMENTS
Atopic dermatitis, or childhood eczema, is characterized by a spreading, sometimes patchy red rash that is itchy, scaly, or blistered. We call it "the itch that rashes" because it starts with itchy skin that disrupts the barrier. When that happens, moisture is lost, and skin becomes dry and more prone to infection. Appearing within the first six months of life, it usually shows up in the folds of the elbows and knees. Children will sometimes even scratch it to the point of bleeding. Atopic dermatitis generally disappears by age twelve. A small percentage of adults continue to suffer from eczema, and it may be localized to areas such as the hands.	Decrease bathing because water can cause further drying of skin Rub soap-free skin cleansers on dry skin and gently towel off without adding water Take antihistamines to treat the itch Apply topical steroids to treat the rash Take antibiotics to treat crusting of infected areas

Seborrheic Dermatitis: When Sebum and Yeast Unite

WHAT IS IT?	TREATMENTS
An inflammatory condition commonly seen in teenagers and adults that is the result of an overgrowth of yeast. Seborrheic dermatitis appears as a greasy, pink scaly rash on the scalp, eyebrows, and crease around the nose. It may be itchy and feel chapped, spreading from the eyebrow area to the cheeks. It frequently flares with stress, cold, dry weather, and the surge of hormones in teens and may be triggered by neurological diseases such as Parkinson's.	Mild topical steroid, a topical sulfur cream, or an anti-yeast cream such as ketoconazole For seborrheic dermatitis of the scalp, zinc, ketoconazole, or tar-containing medicated shampoos

Rosacea: Are You Seeing Red?

WHAT IS IT?	TREATMENTS
Rosacea is a common condition in which the blood vessels of the skin dilate and constrict very easily in response to a whole variety of stimuli including spicy food, alcohol, embarrassment, heat, sunlight, and menopause. Women are more than three times as likely as men to exhibit it, although the symptoms are often more pronounced and severe in men. This chronic skin condition is characterized by intense and frequent flushing or blotchy redness, the appearance of "broken blood vessels" on the cheeks, chin, and nose, and, in some cases, acne-like pimples. It often starts simply as pink, flushed cheeks and eventually evolves into a more permanent redness in the midface, along with pustules and red inflammatory acne-like bumps. See Chapter Eight for more details.	Oral antibiotics, in particular within the tetracycline family, and topical antibiotics such as metronidazole Topical agents such as azelaic acid, benzoyl peroxide, sulfactamide (10%), and sulfur (5%) Pulsed dye laser (PDL) and nonlaser intense pulsed light (IPL) therapies may be utilized by dermatologists Be cautious of glycolic acids or astringents containing alcohol

Caring for Your Sensitive Skin

To heal sensitive skin, you need to repair and strengthen the skin's moisture barrier. Once the moisture barrier is compromised, there tends to be a downward spiral, as increased moisture loss causes a heightened inflammatory response and lessens the skin's ability to self-repair. This, in turn, further increases moisture loss, and the cycle continues.

Thus, step one for recovery is to remove from your regimen anything that could compromise the barrier, such as irritating substances, exfoliation, and peels. Then, you need to provide the skin with ingredients that fill in and repair the barrier, such as dimethicone, allantoin, and lipids. This will allow the skin to heal, keeping moisture in and irritants and microbial agents out.

Minimalism rules: less is more when it comes to caring for sensitive skin. Be gentle with your skin and find products that don't irritate it. If your skin is itchy, treat the underlying itch with an antihistamine. Identify and avoid factors that trigger reactions, such as heat, sunlight, and certain skincare or food products. And remember that nobody knows your skin better than you do. If something isn't working or is making the problem worse, stop using it. Conversely, when you find something that works for your skin, stick with it.

Keep in mind that sensitive skin also reacts to the way it is treated, so don't be too aggressive with your skincare regimen and keep exfoliation to a minimum. Be patient; the odds of finding the regimen that's right for you are in your favor when you are methodical about your approach.

Here are some tips for keeping your sensitive skin looking and feeling its best:

- *Use physical sun blockers such as zinc oxide; avoid chemical sunscreens such as oxycinimate*

- *Avoid hot showers, steam rooms, and sauna baths*

- *Avoid washcloths or loofahs; use only a smooth sponge*

- *Always be gentle when touching skin*

- *Avoid alcohol, propylene glycol, and glycolic acids*

- *Skip toners*

- *Stick with fragrance-free formulas*

- *Find moisturizers that include ceremides, lipids, cholesterol, allantoin, and dimethicone to help repair the skin's sensitive barrier*

- *Look for products containing oatmeal, which may help with itchiness*

- *For itching, take oral antihistimines such as Zyrtec, Claritin, or Benadryl*

- *Apply a thin layer of hypoallergenic moisturizer to skin while it's still moist*

- *Use a humidifier in a dry environment*

- *Do your best not to scratch or rub the skin*

- *Finally, if all else fails, see your dermatologist*

⟩ Are You Making Your Skin Angry?

1. Do you take hot showers or visit steam rooms and sauna baths?

_____ Yes   _____ No

2. Do you use washcloths or loofahs?

_____ Yes   _____ No

3. Do you use products with fragrances?

_____ Yes   _____ No

4. Do you rest your chin in the palm of your hand or touch your face regularly?

_____ Yes   _____ No

If you answered "Yes" to any of the above and you suffer from red, sensitive skin, we recommend you break the habit. These behaviors can make normal skin sensitive and make sensitive skin even more so. Take it easy—your skin will thank you for it!

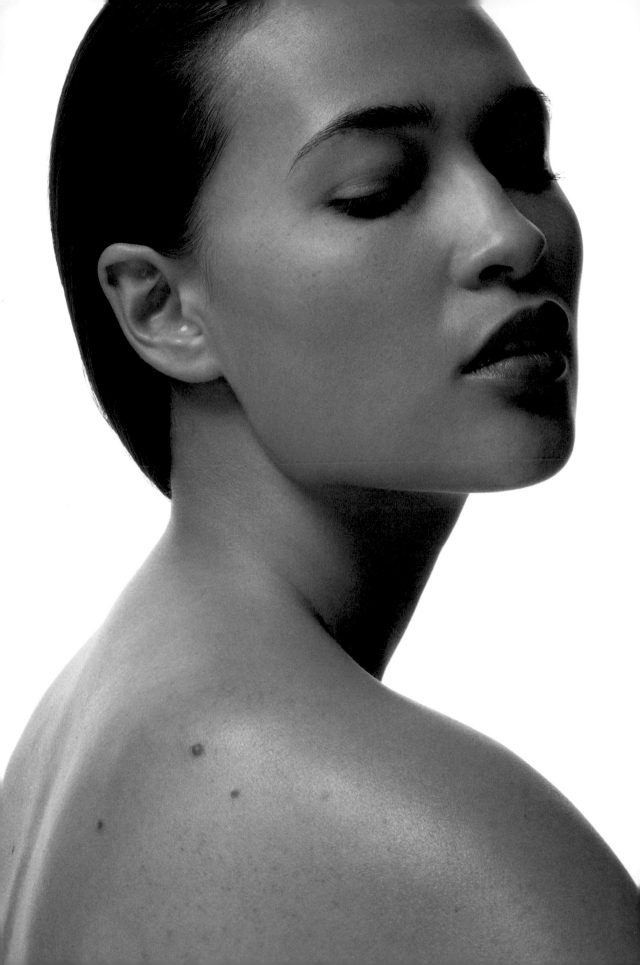

BUMPS AND GROWTHS

And What to Do with Them

11

"What differentiates a beauty mark from an ugly mole? Location, location, location."

Dr. Katie Rodan

Our aesthetic sensibilities find a mole attractive when it is a dark brown, flat, perfectly positioned "beauty mark" adjacent to the upper lip or lower eyelid, as graces the lovely visages of Cindy Crawford and Marilyn Monroe. In the eighteenth century, moles were so highly regarded and coveted that many people often embellished their appearance by cosmetically applying them.

Situated in a less desirable location, a mole is an imperfection, a blemish, something to be dealt with. Recall this scene from *Buffy the Vampire Slayer*:

MERRICK (pulling Buffy's blouse away from her shoulder to reveal the mark of the vampire slayer): "The mark of the coven! The—where's the mark?"

BUFFY: "You mean that big hairy mole? Excuse me: eeyuu. I had it removed."

Sarah Jessica Parker also had her mole, a raised, flesh-colored one, removed from her chin, and it made headlines. So what are you going to do with yours? Cherish it as a sign of distinction, or find yourself a reputable dermatologist to make it disappear?

Before you act in haste, consider what it is you might be excising. The mark on your forehead you detest may represent something entirely different to someone else. For instance, within certain Asian cultures and among Italian folklore, it's said that a beauty mark, particularly on your forehead, means you are very important and extremely loved. As with many things, whom the mark adorns may also change the way it's seen. Take a look at photos of Marilyn Monroe when she was still Norma Jean Baker. Her mole seems to have been "erased" with makeup.

"As a child, this mole on my forehead made me feel self-conscious. Then I traveled to Asia, where I was repeatedly told by the locals that this mark made me special. Now I look at it differently and wouldn't change it for the world."

ERIC, AGE TWENTY-SIX

Ewww: What Is This?

With age, we notice our skin responding to both internal physiological changes as well as our external environment. As it does, a variety of interesting marks and growths start to "visit" various parts of our anatomy, frequently making an unwanted appearance on our face. While these growths are harmless most of the time, they are oftentimes unsightly, and occasionally a new growth might represent a significant health concern. So if there are new growths or any mole changes in size, shape, or color, visit your dermatologist for a skin check. And of course, if anything appears suddenly and is tender or bleeding, book that appointment immediately.

Getting a definitive diagnosis and treatment plan is the key to staying in control of both your appearance and your health. On the following pages, we'll help to demystify many of the most common bumps and growths that we see in our practices or are often asked to examine at cocktail parties. We will provide you with a description of what they look like, why they are there, and what you can do to treat them.

The Mole in the Eye of the Beholder

Those of us with a copious supply of moles may have been surprised during our adolescence when out of nowhere they seemed to appear. Now that they are here, it's important to map them and keep track of their growth and change, because the more moles we have, the greater the risk that one of them will become cancerous.

WHAT YOU SEE

If you're lucky, moles appear as small, pretty brown or black "beauty marks" on your skin. But with age, some "beauty marks" turn ugly, losing their color and protruding like the unsightly, flesh-toned, hairy growths that are associated with the Wicked Witch of the West.

?DID YOU KNOW?

IT IS PERFECTLY SAFE TO PLUCK HAIR GROWING OUT OF A MOLE. THIS WILL NOT CAUSE MULTIPLE HAIRS TO GROW BACK OR STIMULATE CANCEROUS TRANSFORMATION AS PER URBAN MYTH.

WHAT IT IS

In dermatology speak, moles are known as melanocytic nevi and may occur anywhere on the body, being most prevalent on sun-exposed surfaces above the waist. They are generally fewer than five millimeters in diameter (the size of a pencil eraser head), flat or slightly elevated above the surface of the skin, and pigmented or flesh colored. While the vast majority of moles are not dangerous, some can be cancerous, so know your nevi and refer to the ABCDES of melanoma detection (see Chapter Five). Pay especially close attention to a new mole or one whose appearance changes and see a dermatologist for an evaluation.

THE REMEDY

If you don't like the cosmetic appearance of your mole, you have a variety of removal options, most producing little scarring. Moles that protrude from the surface of the skin can be removed with a simple shave biopsy in a dermatology office. This procedure flattens the mole to the level of the surrounding skin. The downside of a shave biopsy is that because the mole hasn't been completely removed, it grows back. However, the trace scar left behind is minimal. Another option for mole removal is a complete surgical excision. This requires stitches and often produces a more obvious linear scar.

Skin Tags

WHAT YOU SEE

A flesh-colored, smooth, hanging piece of skin often found on the eyelids, neck, chest, back, armpits, groin, under the breasts—wherever there are folds of skin. Most skin tags are tiny but if irritated can grow to the size of a pea.

WHAT IT IS

Skin tags (technically known as acrochordons) are benign growths caused by the friction of skin rubbing against skin or clothing. Hormonal changes may stimulate their growth. Some skin tags are involuting moles in the process of disappearing. They tend to be more prevalent in women, particularly after pregnancy, and in middle-aged or elderly people. They are often associated with obesity and can sometimes be mistaken for warts or seborrheic keratoses.

THE REMEDY

A quick snip with a surgical scissor or a quick touch with an electrosurgical spark in a dermatologist's office painlessly removes these skin tags.

Skin Tags: Take Control

A harmless skin tag could signal opportunities for taking control of your health. If it is likely that your skin tags are a by-product of obesity or a hormonal imbalance, caring for the underlying condition will help to prevent recurrence. There is also evidence that people with skin tags have a slightly increased risk of polyps in the colon, so be sure to share your history of skin tags with your internist.

Seborrheic Keratoses

WHAT YOU SEE

Tan, brown, or black growths that look like they have been arbitrarily "stuck on" the skin. The raised edges make them appear almost as if they could be picked off. Cruelly called the "barnacles of old age," they are usually found singularly or in clusters on the face, chest, back, head, and under the breasts.

WHAT IT IS

Often confused with warts or moles, seborrheic keratoses are noncancerous lesions representing excessive growth in the top layer of skin. Since there is a genetic predisposition for seborrheic keratoses, they tend to run in families and are often triggered by pregnancy, estrogen therapy, and age. Because seborrheic keratoses can mimic cancer and cancer can mimic a seborrheic keratosis, it is important to see your dermatologist if you discover a new, solitary lesion. It may need a biopsy.

THE REMEDY

Seborrheic keratoses can be removed easily by a dermatologist with a variety of methods, including surgically shaving them, using liquid nitrogen cryotherapy, or applying intense heat via electrocautery to "melt" them off.

Dermatoses Papulosa Nigra

WHAT YOU SEE

Little black or dark brown bumps, which may grow in clusters, usually appearing on dark skin. Nearly 35% of black-skinned adults in the United States have them. They start out as small freckles under the eyes and on top of the cheekbones (think Morgan Freeman) and tend to increase in size and number with age.

WHAT IT IS

These benign growths begin appearing as small, barely elevated tiny brown spots on the face. Although the cause is unknown, there is a definite genetic relationship, with 50% of those affected having a positive family history. So if your grandmother has them, you're quite likely to get them as well.

THE REMEDY

We most often use electrocautery to lightly burn them off. Make sure your physician is experienced in removing these, because there is a chance of scarring, particularly in darker skin types.

Xanthelasma

WHAT YOU SEE

Soft yellowish bumps or plaques on the mid/upper or lower eyelids. If left untreated, they can get quite large.

WHAT IT IS

These are fat deposits that almost always indicate high cholesterol. In fact, it is quite unusual to get them if you have a healthy lipid level. Therefore, if you have xanthelasma, you should have your cholesterol levels checked by your physician, as they may be a sign of a more serious internal problem.

THE REMEDY

We recommend using carbon dioxide lasers to gently melt these deposits flat. They can also be excised if they are small. Since they appear in the eyelid creases, rarely does their removal leave a visible scar.

Sebaceous Hyperplasia

WHAT YOU SEE

These small, soft yellowish pink bumps become noticeable around middle age (often in the forties and fifties), sprouting up in the oily "T-zone" along the forehead, nose, and cheeks. Usually about the size of a kernel of barley, they are dome shaped with a central depression or pit.

WHAT IT IS

Because sebaceous hyperplasia represents an enlargement of a nonfunctioning singular oil gland, it develops around a central hair follicle. It tends to run in families and often occurs in people who experienced oily complexions as teens. Men are also more prone to these lesions than women.

THE REMEDY

Although it does not pose a medical risk, sebaceous hyperplasia can be cosmetically distressing and will not go away spontaneously. It may be removed by a dermatologist using electrocautery or laser.

Milia

WHAT YOU SEE

Tiny white bumps commonly appearing around the eyes or nose or less frequently elsewhere on the face. They can appear at any age and are often seen on infants.

WHAT IT IS

Milia are small benign cysts that may form for no apparent reason or in response to sun damage, trauma, and possible use of heavy occlusive moisturizers. Contrary to popular belief, they are not calcium deposits and are actually composed primarily of keratin (skin cell) material.

THE REMEDY

Milia that appear during infancy tend to go away spontaneously within a few months. Milia in adults, on the other hand, are chronic and rarely disappear without treatment. The first step in treating milia is to rethink your skincare regimen and discard any heavy products that may be causing the problem. To remove a milium, dermatologists will use a small needle or blade to extract the tiny cyst, which looks like a pearl of thick oil. They can also be treated using microdermabrasion and superficial peels. You may be tempted to just pluck them off yourself, but we don't recommend this because it can cause scarring.

Cherry Angiomas

WHAT YOU SEE

Small red or very dark purple bloodlike bumps on the surface of the skin, especially the torso, that seem to blossom with age.

WHAT IT IS

Appearing spontaneously, usually after forty, cherry angiomas are vascular lesions made up of clusters of tiny dilated capillaries. They are about the size of a pinhead and flat when they first appear, later growing upward of a quarter-inch in diameter and eventually protruding above the skin's surface. While harmless, if traumatized they may profusely bleed.

THE REMEDY

They can be easily removed by electrosurgery or laser vaporization.

Whether you're like Buffy who can't wait to "slay" her mole or like Marilyn Monroe who immortalized hers, knowing what those bumps and growths actually are will help you gain more control over your appearance and your health. And because most of these pesky little nuisances are easily and painlessly removable, they need not occupy center stage on your face. A quick trip to the dermatologist's office and you may forget you ever had them! And so will everyone else.

⊕ Have Your Bumps Checked by a Physician

Most bumps and growths that appear over the course of our lives are harmless, representing only a cosmetic concern. For any new growth, we recommend seeing a dermatologist for an accurate diagnosis and treatment options. Rarely, more serious medical conditions may mimic one of these harmless lesions. Seborrheic keratosis, for example, must be differentiated from melanoma. In the case of cherry angiomas, it is important to be sure they are not actually petechiae, pinpoint red spots often indicative of a low blood platelet count, which may represent a serious medical problem.

> Map Those Moles

Charting the location of your moles annually can help you and your dermatologist track changes and identify cancer early on. Mark up the silhouettes, numbering everywhere you have moles. Make sure to use one color of pen and record the date. For each mole, record detailed information in the chart, referring to the ABCDEs of melanoma from Chapter Five. Do this again in one year with a different color. Make sure to note any new moles or moles that change in shape or color over time.

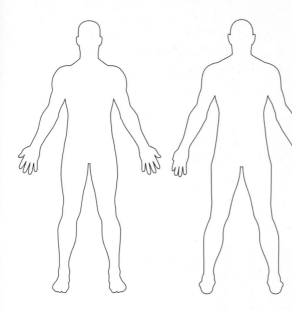

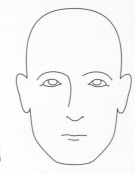

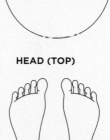

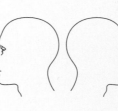

FRONT   **BACK**   **LEFT & RIGHT PROFILE**   **FEET**

FACE   HEAD (TOP)

MOLE #	A—ASYMMETRY Look for spots that aren't symmetrical and that have an odd shape.	B—BORDER Look for a border that isn't sharp and defined.	C—COLOR Look for color that isn't uniform and that has different shades of red, brown, and black.	D—DIAMETER Look for spots the size of a pencil eraser or larger.	E—EVOLUTION Look for spots that change over time.

People with a common genetic condition called dysplastic nevus syndrome may have many more moles than the average person, and these moles are often larger, irregular, or variable in color. Because people with this syndrome have a slightly greater chance of developing melanoma, this exercise is especially helpful for tracking changes in mole size, shape, and color and identifying early skin cancers.

For increased accuracy, you may want to consider photodocumentation of your mole pattern. As needed, share these maps with your dermatologist.

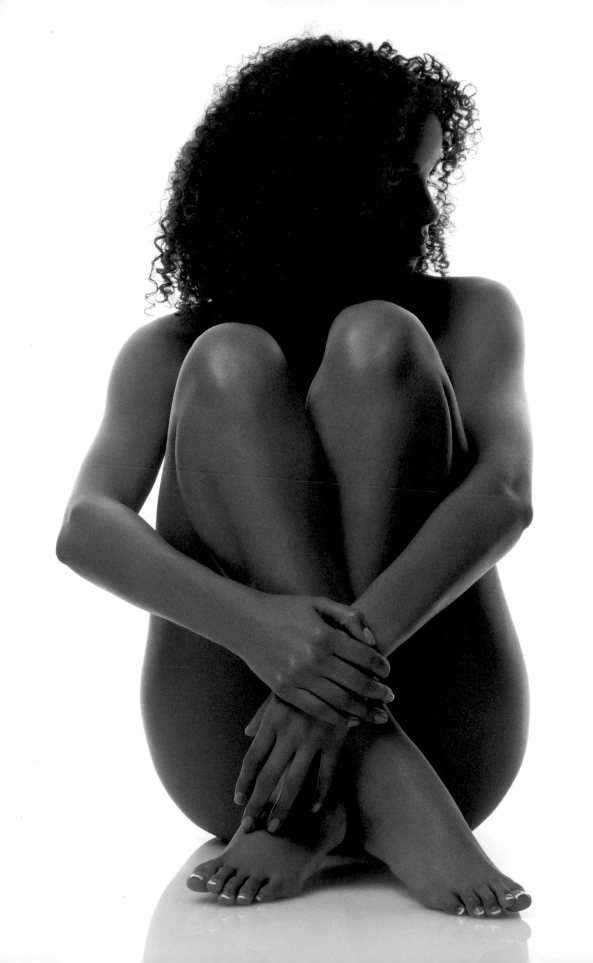

MORE THAN JUST A PRETTY FACE

Looking Great from Head to Toe

12

"Throughout my life, I've always had well-sculpted arms and shoulders, but I rarely wore sleeveless clothes when I was younger. Between the hairiness on my forearms and the ugly red bumps on the back of my upper arms, who would notice the hours I spent at the gym?"

Lori Bush

Have you ever noticed a gorgeous woman who, at first blush, appears to have beautiful skin but upon further observation has a face and hands that seem to belong to different people? Sadly, for all of us, the tremendous effort we put into taking care of our faces may be quickly discounted when our hands, feet, or legs tell a different story. Caring for your skin shouldn't stop at your neck. As dermatologists, our mission is to help you achieve your best healthy-looking skin from the top of your head down to the tips of your toes.

Although we could write an entire book on caring for your hair, nails, and body, in this chapter we've highlighted some of the most common "beyond the face" concerns we hear and offer advice on what you can do to look and feel your best all over.

I lose so much hair when I shampoo that I could make a Barbie doll. Am I going bald?

In terms of investment in appearance, women spend a lot of time and money caring for their hair, a defining aspect of their style, so it's no surprise that the apparent thinning of once thick, luxurious locks is cause for major anxiety.

Female pattern hair loss (FPHL) is not nearly as obvious or well defined as male pattern baldness, although there are those who believe that genetic predisposition resides on the same gene for both women and men. While only 6% of women under age fifty have the hair-thinning characteristics that qualify as FPHL, the incidence increases to 38% by age seventy.

The changes that occur in women's hair are quite different from those in men's, with the first signs of thinning hair being a widening of the part line. The thinner appearance of hair is generally due to diminishing hair density but may be the result of decreased hair diameter as well. In early stages, many women may not even notice that their part line is widening. However, as hair loss advances, the frontal end of the part widens further, presenting with a "Christmas tree" pattern.

For most FPHL, we recommend the use of over-the-counter Minoxidil because it can be very effective in helping you keep more hair on your head. We see the best results with the 5% strength solution. However, because this strength tends to be somewhat greasy on the scalp, we suggest using the 5% solution at night and the 2% strength in the morning. Minoxidil must be used twice a day to be effective, and it may take four to six months to really see the benefits. For women who do not respond to Minoxidil, we sometimes prescribe spironolactone, which suppresses activity of the hormone DHT. For this treatment, it is important that women not be of childbearing age and that serum potassium levels be checked during treatment.

There is also a new laser comb treatment on the market that has been reported to help FPHL, but there have not been convincing clinical trials proving its benefits. And while hair transplantation techniques have improved tremendously and are quite effective for FPHL, very few women elect to go this route.

If hair is lost in patches on other areas of your head, this could be a different dermatological condition, and you should seek the consultation of a dermatologist immediately.

In general, we suggest that you don't stress over what's in the sink but instead keep an eye on that part line.

"When it comes to my female patients, I treat every area of a woman's body as a 'cosmetic unit,' from her face to her back, chest, and even derriere. Every inch of her skin must look great for her to walk with confidence, whether she is wearing an evening gown or a bathing suit."

DR. KATIE RODAN

Hair today, gone tomorrow—will laser hair removal really be the permanent solution I'm looking for? What are the best alternatives for defuzzing my hairy parts?

There are many options for removing unwanted hair. Read on.

LASERS

With lasers created for hair removal, light travels down the dark pigment of the hair and destroys it at the root for semipermanent removal of unwanted hair from the face, nipples, bikini line, armpits, toes, legs, and men's backs. A great benefit is that you do not get the ingrown hairs (or the pain) that often accompany waxing.

However, not everyone is a candidate for laser hair removal. Red, blonde, and gray hair cannot be removed effectively because the laser is attracted to melanin pigmentation. The ideal patient has fair skin with dark hair—think Snow White. Laser hair removal is also not as effective at removing dark hair on dark skin because the laser can't discern where the hair stops and the skin begins. Therefore, the energy required to remove the hair can result in burning and wounding the skin. However, recent breakthroughs allow lasers such as the IPL laser to be adjusted to lower levels in order to remove dark hair on some dark-toned skin.

It may take six to ten treatments scheduled six to eight weeks apart to eliminate hair completely. You cannot pluck hair for one month prior to a laser hair-removal appointment, and you will need some stubble growth in order for the laser to be attracted to the hair. Hair may grow back after a year, although never to the original density, so you may want to return for touch-up treatments.

The cost of treatment depends on the amount of hair you are having removed and can run from $100 for one session on your upper lip to $1,000 for your legs. The procedure can be done by a dermatologist or at a medi-spa. It is one of the most satisfying laser treatments because it is extremely effective with very little discomfort and downtime.

ELECTROLYSIS

If you have red, blonde, or gray hair or very dark skin, you may opt for electrolysis because lasers just won't work on you. Electrolysis requires many more treatments than laser and is a bit more painful. However, it does offer permanent hair reduction. One of the problems is that it can scar, so you need to make sure your technician is not too aggressive with your treatments. For sanitary reasons, make sure the electrologist is using a fresh needle for each client.

WAXING

If you're into torture and spending the majority of your time covering the area with clothing because you are "growing in" the hair, then wax. Here's how it works: you spend four to six weeks letting the hair come in, then wax it off in order to be "hair free" for about a week, only to start the process all over again. You're in a state of stubble more often than not. Additionally, the treatments can be quite painful because you are literally ripping the hair away from your skin.

If you choose to wax, several kinds of waxing methods are available. Sometimes the wax is applied directly to the skin, or sometimes technicians use muslin or linen strips to pull off the hair. Although waxing is safe anywhere on the body, it can cause ingrown hairs, so you may want to soak the area to be waxed in Hibiclens antibacterial liquid soap before and after waxing.

After waxing, you should avoid using Retin-A or strong alpha hydroxy acids in the eyebrow or lip areas, as they can make your skin more sensitive. You may also want to apply a 1% hydrocortisone cream following waxing to soothe the area.

For sanitary reasons, it is important for the technician to use a fresh applicator, usually a wooden tongue depressor, every time he or she puts new wax on you. Make sure he or she doesn't recycle the wax from one client to the next or double dip the tongue depressor, which can transfer infectious agents from your skin to the next person (or worse, allow the person before you to spread bacteria or viral breakouts to you).

SHAVING

Although shaving is the least expensive method of hair removal, it can be the most time-consuming because the hairs grow back so quickly that many people need to shave daily. Shaving can also cause ingrown hairs or folliculitis, little red bumps at the base of the hair, commonly found on the legs and groin. If you are prone to folliculitis, use a new blade each time you shave to lessen the friction against the skin. You may also want to try Hibiclens antibacterial liquid soap on the area; leave this on for a minute prior to shaving. And never leave your razor in a wet, damp shower where it can collect bacteria.

"To help prevent body acne, I tell my patients not to stew in their sweat. In other words, avoid sticky clothing, shower immediately after exercising, and, just as important, use products specifically designed for the body."

DR. KATHY FIELDS

My figure looks great, but the acne on my back is keeping me from wearing that little black dress. Help!

You've invested a lot of sweat equity, and your body is in great shape. Just when you're ready to celebrate with a new swimsuit or backless halter, a pimple derails your plans. It's really not surprising, because many of the elements involved in working out in the first place, such as heat, friction, sweat, and tight clothing, are just the triggers acne needs to thrive. Body acne, particularly on the back, chest, and arms, is surprisingly prevalent. In fact, many facial acne sufferers also experience acne on other body parts. Or, in some cases, you may even suffer from body acne without ever having experienced blemishes on your face.

Although body skin is different from facial skin—it's thicker and denser—the process that causes acne (the plug, the bacteria, the oil, and the inflammation) is the same. However, the appearance of the acne may be very different. For example, you may get a few blackheads and red bumps on your face but deeper, more cystic acne lesions on your back and chest. The acne on the torso is also much more likely to scar. With this in mind, given an exception or two, you should treat body acne the same way you treat blemishes on your face:

- *If you're prone to body acne, treat the entire area daily to heal what's there and prevent new acne from appearing. Spot treatments won't do the job.*

- *Prevent the acne before it appears by avoiding occlusive, nylon, or spandex clothing, which often traps the heat and exacerbates breakouts. After your workout, shower immediately using a medicated cleanser.*

- *Treat blemishes that have surfaced with products that clean pores, reduce oil production, and kill bacteria.*

- Minimize post-acne discolorations with products containing hydroquinone and skin brighteners.

- Use a loofah sponge in the shower to help get to those hard-to-reach places on your torso. Because loofahs can collect bacteria in the warm shower, we recommend that you invest in a rectangular loofah made of cotton that can easily be laundered.

Although benzoyl peroxide is the workhorse ingredient for treating acne, it can also permanently discolor clothing and linens. Therefore, you may want to look for an acne product specifically designed for the body containing salicylic acid as the active ingredient. If your acne is resistant, see a dermatologist because you may need prescription medication.

What are those bumps on the back of my arms? They're driving me crazy!

You're most likely suffering from keratosis pilaris, an extremely common skin disease (nearly 50% of the population suffers from it) characterized by rough, bumpy skin on the upper arms and tops of the thighs. Sometimes referred to as "chicken skin," keratosis pilaris is a build-up of a protein called keratin at the opening of the hair follicle that produces spiky overgrowths of skin that seem to get worse in the winter.

Although you may not like the appearance of these bumps, keratosis pilaris is harmless. At this point, there is no cure, and keratosis pilaris is universally difficult to treat. However, certain treatments may reduce the severity in some people. In some, exfoliation to more quickly renew the skin may be helpful. Additionally, topical retinoids and ammonium lactate cream or lotion that normalizes cell turnover will reduce the textural roughness associated with keratosis pilaris. For more extensive cases of keratosis pilaris, see your dermatologist for a mid-strength topical steroid cream to use on an as-needed basis.

Because keratosis pilaris is so common, there is presently a great deal of clinical research looking for successful therapies. We are confident that more effective treatments will be available in the not-too-distant future.

What can I do to soften rough, scaly patches of skin during the winter?

Some of the symptoms of dry skin are severe roughness, cracking, scaling, and flakiness commonly found on elbows, knees, shins, and hands. The cause of the flakes is the build-up of the uppermost layers of skin (stratum corneum), which have difficulty shedding. In the winter, we turn up the thermostat in our homes' forced-air heating systems, which removes humidity from the air and causes dehydration of our skin. Dry skin is thinner, more fragile, and has less of a protective barrier. Once the skin's barrier is compromised, moisture loss continues, and the skin is vulnerable to the entrance of irritants and infections, often leading to a red, itchy rash.

Does Your Skin Need Psychotherapy?

When skin cells are stressed due to harsh climates or other environmental aggressors, cells go into overdrive and rush to the surface before they are fully mature. The result is increased cell pile-up, creating skin that is uncomfortable, dry, flaky, tight, and irritated. To de-stress your frenzied cells, we like dormins. These plant bulb extracts, found in dormant narcissus bulbs, protect fragile flowers through harsh winters and do the same for our skin, normalizing the lifespan of healthy cells so skin is more resilient to the climate-induced stressors that cause it to feel dry, tight, and generally uncomfortable.

A good way to combat dry skin is to use a mild cleanser without soap or detergents and a moisturizer that contains dormins to help normalize the life span of healthy cells at least once a day. You may even consider using a moisturizing body cleanser that you can apply while you are in the shower. Remember to keep water temperature tepid, not hot, because heat intensifies itching. Moisturize right after your bath or shower when skin is still damp. Additionally, the use of a microdermabrasion paste can help by stimulating exfoliation while leaving behind a protective film.

I had a small wart on my hand, and now I'm noticing a few more. Did I catch them?

Warts, which occur commonly on the hands and the feet, are caused by a viral infection (the human papilloma virus, or HPV) and are moderately contagious, spread by direct or indirect contact (a towel, nail file, etc.) from person to person or from one body part to another. We frequently see warts right around the fingernail or toenail areas that most certainly have been contracted at a nail salon.

Plantar warts are warts located on the soles of the feet and often are quite uncomfortable. The primary method of treatment is to destroy the skin the wart lives in. You can attempt to treat them at home by diligently applying a topical salicylic acid or urea wart treatment every night for several months. We recommend that you first soak your foot to soften the skin and then apply the medication directly to the wart and cover it with a Mediplast plaster you can cut to size. Leave it on overnight, remove it in the morning, and then file away the dead skin with a nail file or pumice stone.

However, make sure you never use this instrument anywhere else, no matter how well you believe you have cleaned it, because you will be spreading the wart virus to other parts of your body. If your home remedies fail, see a dermatologist for liquid nitrogen, laser treatment, electrocauterization, or even surgery to fight this formidable foe.

Help. I have "Grandma hands." How can I make them look as good as my face?

Hands can be a dead giveaway of your age, but if you're like most people, you probably ignore them until the day you look down and notice brown spots, crepiness, prominent vessels, and thin skin.

Just like reversing the discolorations on your face, the key to successfully treating brown spots on your hands is a combination of exfoliation to lift off the dead cells, a system containing lightening and brightening ingredients, and diligent sun protection. A good sunscreen that you apply frequently throughout the day, particularly after you wash your hands, is key. For a little extra protection, you might even consider wearing a pair of sexy driving gloves to block out the UV rays you receive in the car.

For deeper, tougher pigment that won't easily lift, a dermatologist can perform mild peels or laser treatments in conjunction with a topical program. Finally, some women even have fillers such as Radiesse or Sculptra professionally injected into their hands to build up the volume. Just like removing spider and varicose veins on the legs, bulging veins on the back of the hands may be treated by injection sclerotherapy. Remember that like maintaining the most youthful appearance for your face, a little preventative care and protection goes a long way on the backs of your hands. So when you're slathering on the hand cream, look for one that contains sunscreen for daytime use; some even tout brightening and firming ingredients to help keep your hands looking like they're part of the same person as your face.

It seems that as I get older, my nails are chipping and even cracking. Is this normal?

Your nails, which are made up of keratin, are an extension of your skin. With age, your nails naturally become drier, more brittle, and fragile, oftentimes even peeling at the ends. Additionally, you may notice longitudinal linear bands on your nails due to decreased circulation in your fingers. Although this is a normal part of aging, you can minimize these common problems by keeping your hands and nails moisturized and hydrated. Remember that every time you wash your hands or remove nail polish, you are disrupting the protective barrier and dehydrating the skin and nails. Your best defense is to apply a heavy moisturizer to your nails throughout the day, paying particular attention to your cuticles. You may even consider applying a rich treatment such as Aquaphor Healing Ointment at night, which, although too greasy to use during the day, works extremely well to strengthen nails while you sleep.

In general, a healthy cuticle is a healthy nail; it's the seal that protects the nail from irritating or infectious agents. Unfortunately, you and your manicurist may get carried away and attack a cuticle like it's a big weed. This can break the seal, causing damage and infection. So, our advice is to ask your manicurist to either skip or go easy on that part of the treatment to ensure the long-term health of your nails.

"I'm a fan of gel manicures because they last for two weeks. The downside is that if you don't protect your hands from the UV light used to cure the gel, the trade off will be aged, 'old lady hands.' I tell my patients to apply sunscreen, or better yet, do what I do, cut the finger tips off of cotton gloves to shield hands during the curing process."

DR. KATIE RODAN

Are Manicures and Pedicures Safe?

We're not going to make a list of all the horrific infections, fungi, and diseases you can get from getting a manicure or pedicure. Just trust us; it doesn't matter whether you go to the corner nail place or an expensive salon—the sanitation is probably not up to speed, and you're at risk. However, for fewer than fifty dollars, you can make your own nail care kit, with all the tools you need:

- Nail clippers
- Nail file
- Cuticle clipper

- Cuticle pusher
- Nail buffer
- Callous smoother

Purchase these tools at your local beauty supply store and bring them to every appointment. Some salons will even store them for you. This small investment and extra step may save you a later visit to your dermatologist for treatment of nail or skin infections.

Final note: while it may seem the pedicure foot tub offers a blissful moment of zen, it may also be the perfect breeding ground for infectious bacteria. Stainless steel soaks are ideal, but if the salon offers only plastic, make sure it is thoroughly cleaned out with an antibacterial cleanser before you place your feet in it. We want you to be smart and cautious so you can enjoy manicures and pedicures just like we do. You can't be overly cautious. Take a few prudent steps to protect your health; you'll thank us one day.

Do I Have a Foot Fungus, or Are My Feet Just Plain Dry?

If you have dry heels accompanied by white, moist scaling between the toes, chances are you have a fungal infection and will need to use a topical antifungal cream you can get over the counter at the drugstore or through your doctor. To help fight the fungus, keep your feet dry. A great trick is to blow-dry your feet, paying particular attention to the area between your toes. You may also want to pare away the dead skin with a pumice stone. This exfoliation will allow moisturizers and medicines to better penetrate.

For simply dry skin, urea is a great ingredient you can find in many products such as Topix Urix40 Urea Cream or Aqua Care with 10% Urea. A very concentrated lactic acid or glycolic acid moisturizer such as AmLactin Cream is also excellent at relieving dry, cracked feet.

My toenails are discolored and seem to be lifting off my toe. They are so disgusting, I'm embarrassed to wear sandals.

Your nail beds may lift up for a whole variety of reasons, including some medications, infections, or even trauma from hiking or wearing running shoes that are too tight. Once the nail lifts up, it "opens the door" for fungus, bacteria, and yeast to colonize because the moisture, combined with the heat, provides the perfect breeding ground. So if your nail seems to have thickened and turned yellow, white, or blackish green, you most likely have an infection. If you suspect this to be true, see your dermatologist or podiatrist for treatment. And remember that it takes toenails a full year to grow out, so toenail infections require long-term, diligent treatment.

Because of the thickness of toenails, most topical treatments have a difficult time penetrating and are often not successful. The most aggressive treatment for toenail fungus is an oral antifungal medication such as Lamisil, Griseofulvin, or Diflucan. Although quite effective, this treatment can be costly and accompanied by a variety of side effects, so you will need to be monitored by your doctor while taking it. Additionally, there are several home remedies your doctor may recommend. For instance, he or she may suggest applying Clorox bleach with a felt tip applicator to the tip of the infected toenails until the infection clears. Be careful to avoid getting bleach onto skin and unaffected nails. While this can be a successful treatment, it requires several months of diligent daily application.

Nail fungus is tenacious and can spread easily—not only to your other toes but also to your feet. Even if you treat it successfully, it is still likely to return a couple of years later. Keep in mind that the yeasts and fungi that cause nail infections are ubiquitous in the environment. If your immune system is susceptible, these infections will definitely find you. Therefore, prevention is key for long-term maintenance. Once the fungus has cleared, use an antifungal powder daily to prevent it from reappearing. Also keep your feet clean and totally dry; wear flip-flops in public showers, keep running shoes in a cool, dry place when not in use, and make sure you don't keep feet in hot, sweaty socks and shoes.

More Body Questions?

Since your skin is your biggest organ, we're sure we've only scratched the surface regarding the many questions you might have regarding keeping the skin below your neck looking and feeling its best. With that in mind, remember to write down all your questions before you meet with your dermatologist. Many patients don't realize that dermatologists' expertise extends beyond expected skin conditions.

Are You Prepared to Bare?

1. Spring is here. It's all about skirts, dresses, and sandals. When stepping into those flip-flops, you think:

_____ A. Oy! My feet are not flip-flop worthy. Between the scaly heels, the dry feet, and the discolored toenails, I'll stick to tennis shoes.

_____ B. Finally, after a long winter, my feet can breathe.

_____ C. Sandals it is, but wait—what is that smell?

2. It's T-minus one day before you jet-set on your next beach vacation. You grab your bathing suit and immediately:

_____ A. Smile, thinking how excited you are to relax at the beach (in the shade, with sunscreen and a hat, of course).

_____ B. Panic as you notice acne on your chest and back.

_____ C. Go digging for your board shorts to hide the hair growing on your bikini line.

3. The joys of fall: witnessing the leaves changing color, being with family on Thanksgiving, and the occasional warm, sunny day. When you find yourself leaving the sweater behind and opting for a tank top, what comes to mind?

_____ A. Newborn baby: My arms are smooth and sleek, and I can't wait to show them off.

_____ B. Chicken skin: Eeek! Where did all these scaly red bumps come from on the back of my upper arms?

_____ C. My mom: My arms are beginning to look like hers. My summer tan faded but left behind white and brown blotchy skin.

Scoring:

Question 1:	A = -3 points/B = 3 points/C = -2 points
Question 2:	A = 3 points/B = -3 points/C = -3 points
Question 3:	A = 3 points/B = -2 points/C = -3 points

Your Score:

0–9: Great work. You're doing the right things to keep your body looking great, and it should show. Pat yourself on the back and keep up the good work.

-9–0: Don't let your body concerns stop you from showing off your skin. While you have more control over some areas than others, there is always something you can do. You deserve to look as good as you feel from head to toe.

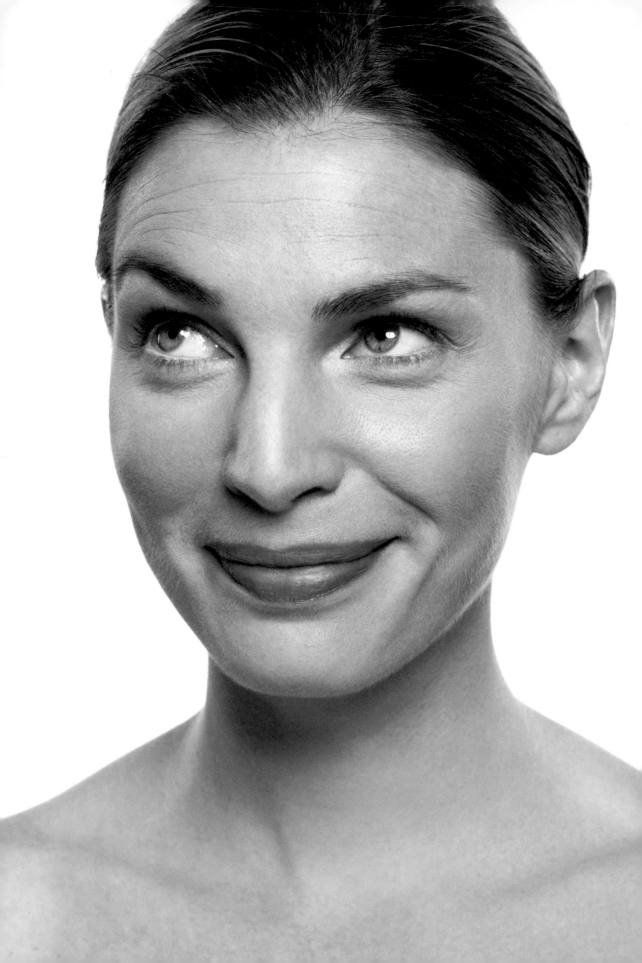

LINES AND WRINKLES

"I'd like to grow very old as slowly as possible."

Author Charles Lamb

13

Renaissance poets and painters established an ideal for fair and spotless beauty that calls for a flawless and radiant complexion from earlobe to earlobe, from the top of the forehead to pink blushing cheeks and red rosebud lips, right down to the crisp edge of the jawline. Writers such as William Shakespeare might have recognized the beauty in imperfection and the wisdom that comes with age, but we continue today to value a complexion unmarred by time and life. Indeed, the pressure to stave off "Father Time" grows ever greater as pop culture proclaims thirty as the new twenty and fifty the new thirty.

When thirty was, well, thirty, you might have expected to start noticing certain visible signs of aging such as a deepening of the "smile" lines trailing between your nose and mouth and the worry creases, those parallel grooves between the eyebrows. It's not fair when these lines of facial expression continue to express themselves even when your face is expressionless. By your forties, wrinkles become more established: the "crow's-feet" around your eyes and the horizontal forehead lines get deeper, while the corners of your mouth start turning down, forming marionette lines that leave you looking either sad or angry.

Then, in your fifties and sixties, crepiness sets in, etching crisscrossing fine lines throughout your once smooth cheeks. All the wrinkles you may have tolerated in your thirties and forties become more deeply etched with each passing birthday. Should we stop there?

Oh, no, there's more. You'll also experience bone, fat, collagen, and elastic tissue loss, causing your face to either sink or sag. This tends to break up the sweeping convex architecture of the youthful face into a series of discrete, concave, angular sections that the human brain recognizes as old. If you are a thin woman with strong, high cheekbones in your thirties, you'll tend to be more of a sinker by your sixties because of the loss of the buccal fat pad, located just below the cheekbone, that results in a hollowed-out appearance.

On the other hand, if you are heavier with a broader face, you'll most likely be a sagger, with jowls replacing your once-defined jawline. Of course, the aging process is a very personal phenomenon, dependant upon everything from genetics to behaviors and habits, including how much time you spend in the sun.

Although aging is inevitable, much of what we consider undesirable is more within our control than people realize. When it comes to the aging face, preventing wrinkles is far easier, less painful, and a lot cheaper than correction.

Today's options for treating wrinkles are numerous and growing, from topical creams and lotions to dermatologic procedures such as laser skin resurfacing, Botox, fillers, and finally, plastic surgery.

Age Progression (Simulated)

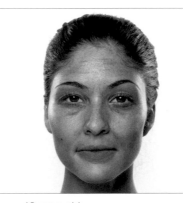 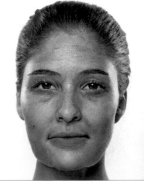

30 years old   40 years old   50+ years old

In the following pages we will briefly discuss the anatomy of a wrinkle and how wrinkles are classified, giving you an overview of treatment options. And in the chapters to follow, we will expand upon the cosmetic options so you can feel great about your appearance at every age.

Characterizing a Wrinkle

When we treat a wrinkle, we first assess its underlying cause. Is it a sleep crease or a line of expression? Was it caused by the sun or by smoking? Its depth, whether superficial or deep, also determines the approach to treatment. The following will explain how we classify wrinkles.

FINE (SUPERFICIAL) WRINKLES

WHAT THEY ARE: Typically caused by sun damage and smoking, both of which accelerate the degeneration of collagen and elastin fibers, these lines are superficial in nature and extend only to the upper dermis. The little lines around the mouth that cause lipstick to bleed are the best example of superficial wrinkles.

WHAT WORKS: Treatments directed at fixing superficial wrinkles must target the upper layers of the dermis. Cosmetic ingredients, by definition, target only the uppermost layer of the skin, the epidermis. Today, we have a better understanding of biofeedback mechanisms that enable the cells in the epidermis to "talk to" cells in deeper tissue layers, causing a specific response such as building collagen. We believe this mechanism explains why we are seeing impressive outcomes with topically applied antiaging peptides.

Topical treatment is the simplest approach for treating these fine wrinkles and the best place to start preventing new ones from forming.

DEEP WRINKLES

WHAT THEY ARE: Caused by the degradation of the structural components of the skin, including elastin, collagen, and fat, deep wrinkles extend through the upper dermis into the mid dermis and lower dermis. The loss of fat cells beneath the wrinkle coupled with lax connective tissue above it means wrinkling and sagging eventually go hand in hand. A droopy mouth is a perfect example.

WHAT WORKS: Deep wrinkles require fillers that are designed to replace the volume that has been lost. Restylane is a volumizing filler that is very effective for lessening the "parentheses" formed by deep nasolabial folds. We will take a more in-depth look at volumizing fillers in Chapter Sixteen.

"Each one of us reacts in a personal way to our own aging face. I never want to impose my own standards of beauty on another person. That's why every patient of mine is handed a mirror and asked to point out specifically what bothers her, and then we take it from there."

DR. KATIE RODAN

?DID YOU KNOW?

SLEEPING ON YOUR BACK COULD BE BETTER THAN BOTOX. SUZANNE IS A PATIENT WHO HAD DEEP LINES THAT SHE WANTED TO ELIMINATE WITH BOTOX. SHE HAD NO CLUE HER SLEEPING POSITION WAS THE CAUSE OF HER "WRINKLES." SLEEPING ON HER BACK WAS THE SIMPLE AND COST-FREE SOLUTION.

DYNAMIC WRINKLES

WHAT THEY ARE: A dynamic wrinkle is caused by muscle movement. The forehead frown lines, those two parallel creases making the number eleven between your eyebrows, result from the repetitive contraction of three muscles, two corrugaters and one procerus, tugging against the skin above and eventually engraving wrinkles.

WHAT WORKS: Botulinum toxin, better known as Botox Cosmetic or Reloxin, inhibits muscle activity, allowing a relaxation of the skin and a disappearance of the wrinkle. It's truly amazing how erasing these creases can transform your face. It makes you look happier and more relaxed and often changes the way people respond to you.

STATIC WRINKLES

WHAT THEY ARE: In contrast to wrinkles seen when muscles contract, static wrinkles are evident when the facial muscles are at rest. The most distressing static wrinkles tend to be those that occur where the lower area of the eye socket meets the top of the cheekbone, sometimes known as "tear troughs." Static wrinkles are the most difficult to treat, but when they are correctly addressed, the improvement in appearance can be quite impressive.

WHAT WORKS: Not treatable with botulinum toxin, static wrinkles require fillers to replace lost volume. Microdermabrasion procedures may also help to build collagen because the pull of the vacuum on the skin may stimulate collagen growth. But the reality is that if you have significant wrinkling and a hollowed, gaunt face, you will likely need a long-lasting, deeper filler to dramatically improve facial wasting.

Stacking the Deck

Our philosophy of antiaging treatments is based on the power of combination therapy. Many options are available to treat the aging face: moisturizing creams with active cosmetic ingredients such as peptides, alpha hydroxy acids, antioxidants, and sunscreen; medicated treatments such as retinoids; cosmetic procedures including peels, microdermabrasion, laser resurfacing, fillers, and Botox; and finally, plastic surgery. Taken together, these treatments are synergistic, maximizing the outcomes and longevity of benefits.

At the end of the day, the best wrinkle is the one you never get. Decide today how you want to look tomorrow. Treat your skin before wrinkles make an unwanted appearance on your face. Here's our spin on the old saying: an ounce of prevention is worth a pound of filler.

⇨ Assess Your Wrinkles

Not all wrinkles are created equally.
Take a few moments to assess your wrinkles and discover how to best minimize them.

1. Describe your relationship with foundation.
_____ A. I never use foundation.
_____ B. I use some foundation.
_____ C. I use heavy foundation.
_____ D. I am unable to use foundation because it cracks on my skin.

2. Look at your face in the mirror. Do you see:
_____ A. Very few or no lines and wrinkles, with an even skin tone.
_____ B. Minor wrinkles associated with movement. Perhaps when you smile you have crow's-feet, or when you frown you get "11s," or when you drink from a straw you see lip lines. Regardless of location, these all go away once you release the expression.
_____ C. Wrinkles that are worsened by contraction of facial muscles (smiling, frowning) but that are still visible even after the expression is gone from your face.
_____ D. Wrinkles throughout your face, such as parentheses (nasolabial folds), tear troughs, and marionette lines along the lower part of the jaw.

3. How is your skin texture and elasticity?
_____ A. Skin is firm and smooth.
_____ B. Skin is showing some signs of roughness but snaps back into place after it is pulled or stretched.
_____ C. Skin is red and ruddy.
_____ D. Skin is rough and has lost its bounce and "snap-back" ability.

4. Do you have enlarged pores on your face?
_____ A. No.
_____ B. They are slightly larger than when I was younger; however, they are not very noticeable.
_____ C. Yes.
_____ D. Yes, my pores are significantly larger than when I was in my twenties, thirties, and forties.

Scoring:

If you answered mostly As: At this point, you don't really have wrinkles. The absolute best thing you can do to keep your skin looking great is to wear broad-spectrum sunscreen (zinc oxide or avobenzone). We can't say it enough. Your skin will thank you. You may also want to consider using moisturizers and/or over-the-counter lotions containing alpha hydroxy and antioxidants.

If you answered mostly Bs: You are prone to developing mechanical or dynamic wrinkles. Changing your habits and daily preventative skincare can go a long way. Make sure to protect your skin daily with broad-spectrum sunscreen (zinc oxide or avobenzone) and start sleeping on your back, wearing sunglasses, and avoiding straws. A daily program of exfoliation and active cosmetics such as peptides or retinol along with diligent sun protection will help keep those dynamic wrinkles from becoming etched into your skin. You may also consider Botox in the appropriate areas so that your repetitive facial movements don't cause static wrinkles.

If you answered mostly Cs: You have wrinkles and skin changes cause by the environment. In addition to protecting your skin daily with broad-spectrum sunscreen (zinc oxide or avobenzone), you will want to incorporate a daily program of exfoliation, a topical skin-brightening treatment, and broad-spectrum sunscreen to reduce skin discolorations. You may also want to consider nonablative laser resurfacing, mild chemical peels, microdermabrasion, fillers, and Botox.

If you answered mostly Ds: You have wrinkles and skin changes cause by biology. In addition to protecting your skin daily with broad-spectrum sunscreen (zinc oxide or avobenzone), you may consider fractionated CO_2 lasers, fillers, and Botox to improve the look of your skin.

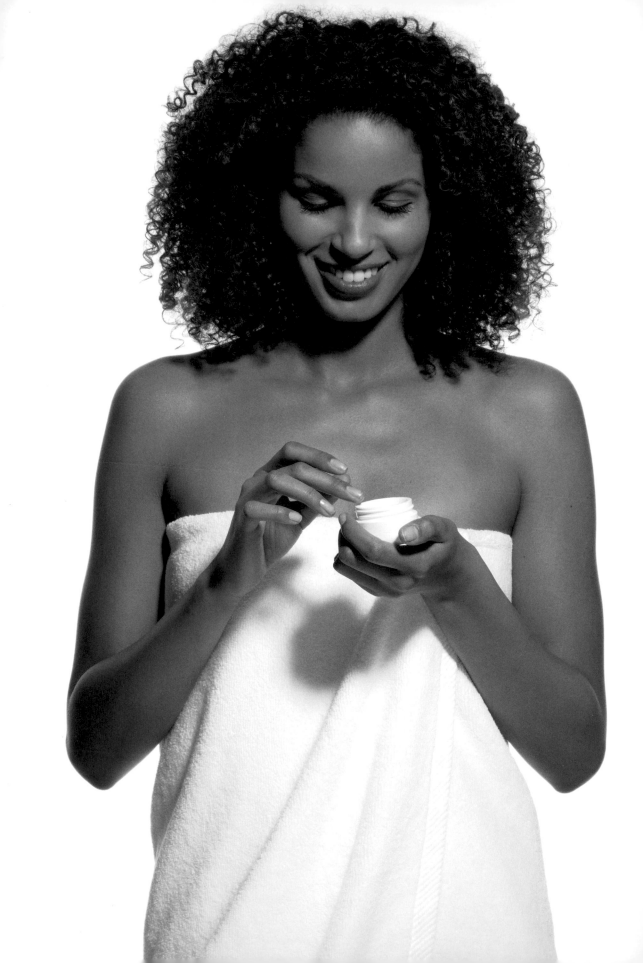

DAILY
TREATMENTS
For Skin Longevity

14

"When it comes to lines and wrinkles, the sooner you start prevention, the later you'll start correction."

Dr. Kathy Fields

Although there is no such thing as a "face-lift in a jar," certain products available today can effectively prevent and reverse revealing signs of skin aging. A pivotal point in skincare occurred in the mid-1980s. Prior to that time, topical skincare for aging was basically tied to maintaining or restoring skin hydration, avoiding harsh, lipid-stripping cleansers, and applying moisturizers with humectant properties to the skin.

That all changed as dermatologists began observing some unexpected outcomes with their adult acne patients who were being treated with a topical vitamin A derivative, a retinoid-based drug call Retin-A. In addition to clearing acne, patients using Retin-A began observing improvement in the signs of skin aging. They saw reduction in superficial lines and wrinkles, improvement in skin texture, and refinement of pores. And although the FDA had approved the drug only for acne, word spread quickly about the prescription wrinkle cream that really worked.

The cosmetic industry reacted instantly, investigating other areas of medical science to identify potentially new ingredients and technology that could be utilized in advanced skincare. The category that today is often referred to as "cosmeceuticals" was born.

Complexities of Complexion Perfection

Aging is a complex phenomenon. As we grow older, our skin's inherent antiaging mechanisms diminish: defenses weaken, critical processes slow, and the rate of breakdown accelerates. A daily regimen needs to replenish or restore what's lacking and prevent or interrupt aging processes.

In addition to reinforcing skin's defenses with a daily application of sunscreen, an antiaging regimen should rejuvenate the skin's surface, restoring elasticity, supporting natural collagen production, and decreasing the appearance of wrinkles. Here's a quick look at the spectrum of benefits a good antiaging regimen should deliver:

- *increased epidermal cell turnover*

- *normalized cells in the epidermis*

- *a compact, smooth stratum corneum*

- *refined pores*

- *resiliency to environmental damage*

- *interruption of collagen and elastin breakdown associated with environmental damage and inflammation*

- *signaling of natural collagen synthesis*

Pharmaceutical Science Creates Today's New Skincare Options

There are dozens if not hundreds of new ingredients introduced every year for treating the signs of skin aging. In our experience both as dermatologists and as skincare developers, very few make the transition from "promising" to "proven" to a dermatological "staple." In the following paragraphs, we'll briefly discuss the pharmaceutical background of key active cosmetic ingredients and highlight those we find the most beneficial or that show the most promise in preventing and correcting the signs of skin aging.

RETINOIDS

PHARMACEUTICAL ORIGIN: Treatment of acne and psoriasis

APPLICATION TO AGING: Because treatment of acne and psoriasis involves the normalization of the skin's keratinization process (the formation and life cycle of normal healthy skin cells), retinoids have been studied extensively for their ability to support the skin's natural cellular renewal processes. Additional research specifically applied to aging has shown that retinoids can block the accelerated rate of collagen breakdown in skin that results from enzymes called MMPs (or matrix metalloproteinases).

A pharmaceutical retinoid may be obtained as the prescription drug tretinoin under the brand names Retin-A or Renova. The most effective cosmetic retinoid is retinol, which may be obtained without a prescription in a variety of skincare formulations.

Since their first use for cosmetic application in the 1980s, retinoids have played a key role in advancing options in daily antiaging skincare. However, retinoids should be used judiciously since, by nature, they can be irritating, causing skin to become red, dry, and inflamed.

HYRDOXY ACIDS

PHARMACEUTICAL ORIGIN: Treatment of scaling skin conditions

APPLICATION TO AGING: Like treatment of severely scaling skin conditions, aging skin requires help in the release of dead skin cell buildup to create a healthier skin surface. Hydroxy acids effectively loosen desmosomes, the junctions between cells, helping skin more effectively shed desiccated epidermal cells to create a smoother, more compact surface and retain moisture more efficiently. Therefore, hydroxy acids have become an important group of skincare ingredients for their role in promoting vital skin cell turnover. Used in lower concentrations, hydroxy acids such as lactic, glycolic, or lactobionic acid are appropriate for home use on a daily basis. Of note, however, is that a large percentage of the population may experience sensory irritation (stinging) when first using alpha hydroxy acids. By starting slowly, with intermittent use in the first couple of weeks, most people will find that their skin accommodates and the stinging greatly diminishes or disappears completely.

> "How do I get my fifty-three-year-old skin to behave like my nineteen-year-old daughter's and renew itself every twenty-eight days instead of every sixty days? Simple—exfoliation! Kick out the old cells and bring in the new."
>
> **DR. KATIE RODAN**

PEPTIDES

PHARMACEUTICAL ORIGIN: Wound healing

APPLICATION TO AGING: Skin's inherent regenerative and repair processes involve naturally occurring proteins called peptides. Peptides are involved in virtually all natural biological processes and are one of the body's key mechanisms for cellular communication, signaling the start of cellular processes or, conversely, blocking undesirable processes. When there is trauma or damage to the skin, specific peptides trigger and enable the repair or healing processes. By creating skincare peptides that follow the same amino acid sequences as naturally occurring peptides, skin cells can be "signaled" to initiate natural collagen production and other restorative processes. Optimally sequenced peptides have very little potential to cause irritation or allergic responses and have become a key area of skin science research. Peptides are, however, extremely expensive, costing

What about Pores?

The universal complaint in our office for the over-thirty crowd is "I hate my pores." As we get older, our pores appear larger, and that is just a fact of life. Here's why. Pores are surrounded by collagen fibers. With age, as collagen production slows and collagen breakdown accelerates, pores lose support, flatten out, and widen.

Another factor that impacts the size and appearance of pores is the pile-up of dead skin cells.

What works? Poly hydroxy acids gently desquamate the cell pile-up in the pores. As you age, retinoids and peptides help increase collagen production, which keeps pores looking smaller. Additionally, salicylic acid peels and microdermabrasian help.

up to ten thousand times more than a typical skincare ingredient, so formulations that contain the required concentration for optimal benefits can be quite pricey.

Taking a Page out of Nutritional Science

Another important source of antiaging active cosmetics comes from the area of nutritional science. Throughout the world, the way skin ages can often be correlated to local diets. While many nutrients that benefit the skin are best obtained through diet, topically applied nutrients, particularly certain key antioxidants, can help reinforce skin's natural defenses against collagen breakdown and other aging effects associated with free radical activity or oxidative stress. Vitamins C, E, and CoQ10 are well recognized as part of skin's antioxidant network and are now being joined by a host of new antioxidant options for skincare.

Active Cosmetics in Antiaging Skincare

INGREDIENT	MECHANISM OF ACTION	EXPECTED BENEFIT
Polyethylene (microdermabrasion) grains	Sloughing dead layer of stratum corneum to signal upregulation of collagen production	Smoothing of skin surface and softening of fine (superficial) wrinkles
Hydroxy acids (glycolic, lactic, salicylic acid)	Normalizing desquamation (cell turnover) and cell renewal for compact stratum corneum and unplugging pores	Smoothing of skin surface, softening of fine (superficial) wrinkles, and minimizing the appearance of enlarged pores
Antioxidants (vitamin C, green tea, Idebenone, etc.)	Protecting against collagen and elastin breakdown associated with free radical damage	Reversing sallow complexion and preventing fine (superficial) wrinkles
Retinoids	Blocking collagen breakdown and improving cell renewal	Reducing fine (superficial) wrinkles, improving skin elasticity, brightening skin, and minimizing appearance of enlarged pores
Matrix-building peptides	Depending on amino acid sequence, boosting collagen production and supporting skin's structural matrix	Softening of fine (superficial) wrinkles and firming of skin surface

Are You Skincare Agnostic?

If you've been sitting on the sidelines trying to decide whether you buy all the hype about skincare, you're in for a very pleasant surprise. Virtually every clinical study we have conducted as skincare product developers has demonstrated that those basic soap-and-water loyalists almost always see a dramatic difference in the quality of their skin once they step up their game with modern skincare technology.

Make a Daily Investment in Your Skin's Future

Worrying about those wrinkles that have yet to appear won't keep them from forming; in fact, worrying will accelerate their formation. Instead, take positive action by incorporating a regimen of intelligent skincare into your daily routine. And if you have or are considering investing in a cosmetic procedure, protect that investment with a solid program of daily skincare. Here's what we recommend for all our skin rejuvenation patients:

"The first antiaging product you should buy is the right sunscreen with UVA/UVB protection."

DR. KATHY FIELDS

Use a broad-spectrum UVA/UVB sunscreen every day. You may also want to find a moisturizer containing SPF for two-in-one benefits.

Use products containing retinoids (such as retinol or tretinoin) to reduce winkles, improve elasticity, and even improve skin color.

Strategically incorporate antiaging peptides into your routine. There are a growing number of benefits that can be achieved with these small-chain amino acids that communicate a specific action for cells to take. Importantly, peptides used in skincare formulations have a lower risk of irritation than many of the other active cosmetics and, in some cases, actually block inflammation on the skin. This makes them a good option when skin sensitivity is of concern.

Look for products that incorporate tried-and-true alpha hydroxy acids. AHAs improve skin texture and reduce the signs of aging by increasing collagen density, enhancing epidermal shedding, and fading surface discolorations. Poly hydroxy acids are potential alternatives to alpha hydroxy acids, as they may be used in higher concentrations without causing as much stinging as AHAs.

Incorporate products containing antioxidants. These intervene at different levels to protect the skin against damaging free radicals. Specifically:

- *Vitamin C stimulates cell renewal and promotes collagen formation, which may reduce wrinkles, thicken skin, and protect against sun damage*

- *Vitamin E neutralizes free radicals that threaten healthy skin*

- *Other common antioxidants include green tea, Resveratrol, CoQ10, coffee berry, Idebenone, and soy, to name a few*

When to Start

Start now. No matter how old you are, today is not too soon (or too late) to start ensuring a healthy, youthful-looking future for your skin. If you have children, you're teaching them about protecting their skin's future by using sunscreen. If you're a young adult and your acne or other skin concerns are under control, you can start incorporating active antiaging cosmetics into your routine to keep your skin looking its youthful best into your thirties, forties, and beyond. And if you've seen your fortieth birthday come and go, antiaging skincare can help compensate for the changes associated with the passing of time and promise that ninety will be a beautiful birthday, too.

Avoid disappointment by understanding that topical daily skincare products, no matter how advanced, are treating changes occurring only on the top layers of skin. And while they can work wonders to help your skin look its best on a daily basis and slow the aging process through the years, no cream is going to replace your fat pads or the bone loss you experience with age. We can all hope that these signs of aging will one day also be addressed through a magic lotion or potion, but for now, at least there are lasers, fillers, and other dermatological advances to pick up where daily skincare leaves off. Read on ...

Lines and Wrinkles—
What You Can Address Topically

Wrinkle-Forming Habits

	Sometimes	Always	Never
Do you:			
1. Drink from a straw?	_____	_____	_____
2. Wear sunglasses?	_____	_____	_____
3. Sleep on your side?	_____	_____	_____
4. Fluctuate in weight +/- 10 lbs?	_____	_____	_____

Scoring:

Question 1: Sometimes = -1   Always = -2   Never = +2
Question 2: Sometimes = +1   Always =+2   Never = -2
Question 3: Sometimes = -1   Always = -2   Never = +2
Question 4: Sometimes = 0   Always = -2   Never = +2

Your Score:

6-8 points: Forever young! Whether you know it or not, you are taking extra steps to ensure your skin looks younger than its years. Keep up the great work.

3-6 points: Time is on your side—but not forever. Incorporate more good habits into your routine today to keep your skin looking its best for years to come.

0-3 points: You may be young at heart, but don't take your looks for granted. Push yourself to incorporate as many of these positive behaviors as possible to help keep your skin looking great for as long as possible.

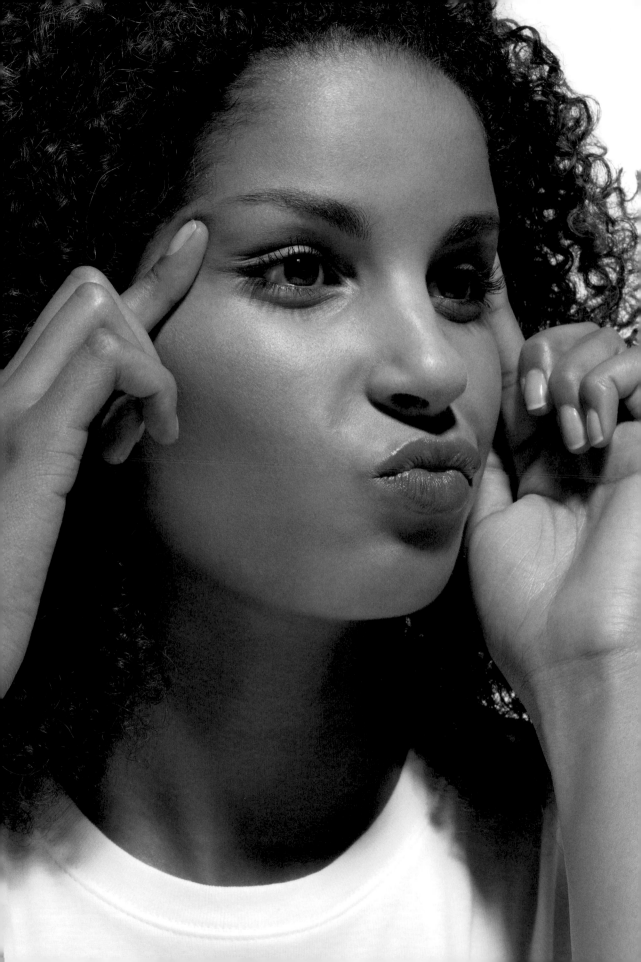

REJUVENATION BY APPOINTMENT

Is It Right for You?

15

"Women are not forgiven for aging. Bob Redford's lines of
 distinction are my old age wrinkles."

Jane Fonda

E ach of us has our own way of dealing with aging. Some of us are fatalistic: nature giveth and nature taketh away—que sera sera. Most of us take personal pride in an appearance that reflects a healthy lifestyle, embracing every change that comes with the natural aging process. And there's a smaller percentage of us who put up more of a fight, feeling no remorse over "fooling Mother Nature."

A Personal Decision

Individual reasons for taking a more aggressive approach to facial rejuvenation are as varied as the rejuvenation procedures themselves. For some, it may be a perceived job requirement. Self-confidence in one's appearance can impact effectiveness in business negotiations, court appearances, and countless other career situations. For others, a rapid and major improvement in appearance can offer a new lease on life when dealing with major personal events such as a divorce or a job change. And for some, it's simply about feeling happy with the reflection in the mirror. All of these reasons are valid, provided decisions are based on a clear understanding of the risks and benefits of the treatments, the skill of the practitioner, and realistic expectations.

Where to Start

Cosmetic dermatology has been called "the fastest-growing segment of the medical industry," with more than nine billion dollars spent annually on cosmetic procedures. So, in the following chapters, we want to give you a peek behind the curtain at what is going on in the progressive world of aesthetic medicine. Our intent is not to convince you or even suggest that a procedure is right for you. Rather, we want to educate you and share our observations about and experiences with the options that are not only available today but also on the horizon.

Be Proactively Involved in Your Treatment

Our advice to those ready to consider an aesthetic procedure is to take the same approach you would if you were seeking treatment for a medical condition. Consider first what you want to change about your appearance, and then seek a specialist who can offer advice and a range of options for achieving the best possible result. Avoid scheduling your cosmetic procedure as if you were ordering from a take-out menu. There are numerous clinics willing to perform an expensive procedure for anyone with the financial means, even if it's not the ideal solution for you.

It's also important to research the training and experience of your practitioner in the area of aesthetic medicine. Because these aesthetic procedures are financially lucrative, there are many doctors besides dermatologists and plastic surgeons (even dentists, nurses, and aestheticians) with very little training who are performing laser treatment and Botox. That is not to say there isn't some outstanding work being done by ER doctors, ob-gyns, pediatricians, and nurse practitioners. However, we strongly advise seeking references when your face is at stake.

Today there are a wide array of quick-fix nonsurgical treatments available that can dramatically improve your appearance by softening lines and wrinkles, plumping facial contours, helping control skin conditions, and removing unwanted growths and marks. In some instances, these treatments can offer a less invasive and safer alternative to going under the knife. Often, the benefit of one procedure or technique is complemented or enhanced by another, so multiple or repeated treatments are often required to achieve the optimal results.

In the following chapter, we'll discuss the most popular procedures performed in our offices. Additionally, we'll provide information about options you may want to investigate but that we have not adopted because they are either too risky or still somewhat experimental, requiring additional clinical testing to be proven truly safe and effective.

If It Sounds too Good to Be True...

As you explore the options in this book and beyond, keep in mind that new aesthetic "miracles" enter the market every couple of years with claims that compare them to face-lifts without surgery. There have been a great many investment dollars poured into the development of new aesthetic technology, and this technology is being launched at a fast pace with pressure on manufacturers to get to market quickly. Therefore, new devices are often publicized to the consumer before medical practitioners have had a chance to properly evaluate them. The touted benefits are often over-promised and underdelivered. And even when the new technology is indeed the next big thing, it may take doctors a year or longer to optimize their techniques and work through the procedural nuances and instrumentation settings to obtain the desired and safe results.

Frequently, new devices pop up on the radar and are popular for a short time, only to be replaced by the next fad. The risk for you is that if you are one of the first patients of a doctor who is an early adopter of the new procedure, you are essentially an experiment. Diligent research on your part is also prudent, as all of these new rejuvenation devices are expensive and represent a major capital investment for the practitioners who acquire them. Because there can be an overriding financial interest in performing procedures that are still experimental or already considered passé or inef-fective, it is well worth your time to know what is deemed current, proven, and state-of-the-art.

Bottom line: don't be a guinea pig by being too early. But don't forgo the best possible results by missing out on the incredible and proven advancements in treatment options available today. If you are investing your money, invest the time in doing the research, too. The results will be worth it.

▷ Are You Ready for Cosmetic Procedures?

Is it time for Botox, or any other cosmetic procedure for that matter? We ask our patients a few simple but important questions when they are considering a procedure:

1. Does the problem affect how you feel about yourself? _____
   _____

2. Does the problem impact how you interact with others? _____
   _____

3. Have you tried topical products to address the problem? _____
   _____

4. Assuming that you are happy with the outcome, are you committed to maintenance
   (usually every four to twelve months)? _____
   _____

5. Have you researched potential side effects, and are you confident that the benefits
   outweigh the risks? _____
   _____

If you answered "Yes" to all of the above, schedule your cosmetic procedure today. If not, we recommend you do some additional research and/or introspection before moving forward. Years in private practice have taught us that for best results, patients need to be ready, educated, and committed.

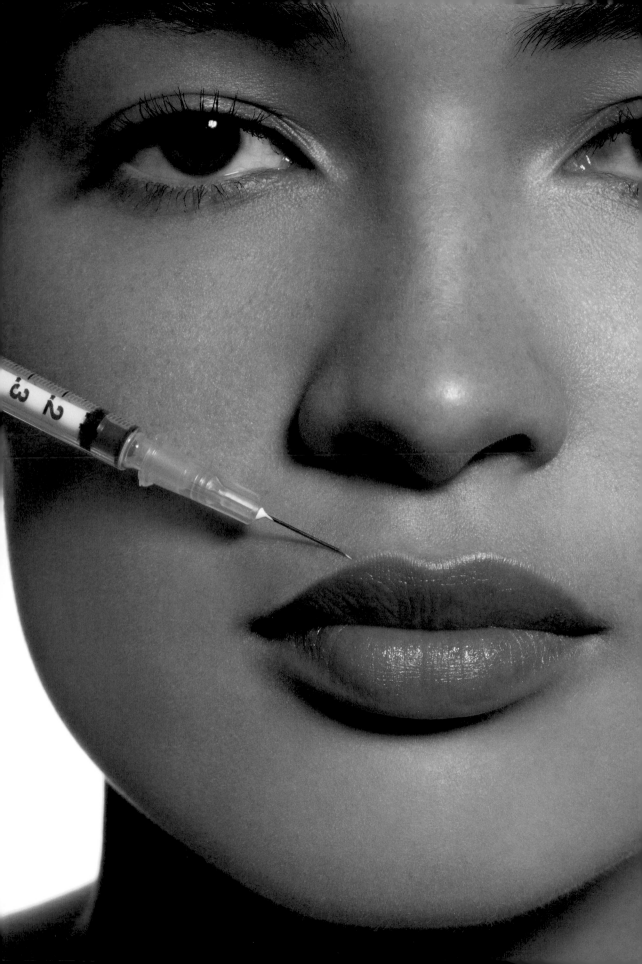

INTERVENTION

Options for the Aging Face

"I joined Facebook at age fifty-two and posted a recent photo of myself. Friends from high school and college have found me and commented about how great I look. That alone makes every nickel I've spent on filler injections worth it!"

Teri, age fifty-three

Through our thirties and into our forties, diligent sun protection and adherence to the appropriate topical regimen can help to stave off many of the hallmarks of the aging face. But sooner or later, the architecture of the skin and its underlying support structure begin to change at a rate faster, and in ways that are more profound, than our preventative and home-based treatments can counter. These changes generally fall into one of three categories: decreased collagen production, dynamic tissue breakdown, or loss of volume. Today, many options exist to address each or all of these changes in skin and shift the aging paradigm with the help of an experienced cosmetic dermatologist.

> "Microdermabrasion is for more than just wrinkles. I had a five-year-old patient who fell on the playground and had a deep cut on her forehead. We started weekly treatments of painless microdermabrasion right away, and her scar is completely gone. She has a friend who also fell and cut her forehead but didn't receive microdermabrasion. After several years, this young girl continues to have a very visible permanent and psychologically damaging scar. Her parents are waiting for her to grow up before they have it treated. It is important to let everyone know that we can fix those scars right away."
>
> **DR. KATHY FIELDS**

Skin Resurfacing

Facial skin resurfacing can be traced to the ancient Egyptians who applied abrasive masks of alabaster particles to their skin. When Cleopatra's beauty routine involved coating her skin with sour milk, little did she know she was applying a source of alpha hydroxy acids (AHA) that, thousands of years later, would be an antiaging skincare staple.

Since these early times, various substances and techniques have been used to peel or resurface the skin, including acids, minerals, plants, and sandpaper-like materials (not to mention sandpaper itself—straight from 3M). The value of these treatments is rapid exfoliation at varying depths, depending upon how deep the treatment must be for a desired benefit. The most common methods of superficial skin resurfacing today are microdermabrasion and glycolic peels, which improve skin texture and tone.

Because many of these procedures can be performed at any corner salon, it is important to select a location with a trained aesthetician, nurse practitioner, or dermatologist. It is crucial that the professional performing the procedure selects the right procedure for the right patient. This will guarantee the best results and the least complicated recovery. In some cases, more aggressive microdermabrasion may be performed by a dermatologist to treat surgical or traumatic scars. Although the credentials required to perform these services are regulated state by state, for more serious matters, make sure you have the procedure performed by a trusted dermatologist.

Red-Carpet Ready

If you are heading down the red carpet in a few days or have some spectacular event to attend, opt for microdermabrasion rather than a peel. Remember Samantha Jones' reaction to a chemical peel in *Sex and the City*? You don't want to hide under a dark black veil during an important premiere moment!

Superficial Resurfacing Procedures

PROCEDURE	Hydroxy Acid Peel	Microdermabrasion
WHAT IT IS	Light peel, most commonly with salicylic or glycolic acid. Exfoliates, enhances cell renewal, and increases penetration and potency of other topical agents.	Abrasion of superficial layers of the skin to remove dead surface cells and enhance cell turnover.
HOW IT'S DONE	Acid is applied evenly on face and neck and left on several minutes until a white film or "frost" develops. Acid is then neutralized with alkaline solution or washed off.	Two primary methods: 1. Fine crystals of aluminum or sodium bicarbonate are sprayed onto the skin at a precise pressure and then concurrently vacuumed off with adjustable intensity of suction. 2. A rough-textured handheld instrument is applied to the skin for abrasion. This is followed immediately with suction to remove exfoliated cells.
TOUTED BENEFITS	Helps clear acne, refine pores, improve texture, and diminish signs of sun damage.	Smoothes skin's surface, refines pores, brightens skin, and stimulates collagen and elastin growth, helping diminish the appearance of superficial marks.
RISKS	For darker skin types, irritation may lead to post-inflammatory hyperpigmentation.	Very minimal when care is taken to protect the eyes. Less risk of hyperpigmentation than with peels.
HOW MANY YOU NEED	Performed every other week for a minimum series of five to six, then monthly to help maintain benefits.	Performed every week for a minimum series of five or six, then monthly to help maintain benefits.
COST	$120–$180 per session	$120–$180 per session
DISCOMFORT/ DOWNTIME	Minimal: tingling, burning, or stinging. Minor "pinkness" for up to forty-eight hours. May lightly peel on third day.	Little to no discomfort or downtime. Often described as feeling like a "cat licking your face." Skin may feel tight after procedure.
OUR RATING	Good when similar results can't be achieved with self-treatment. Boosts results of an at-home treatment program.	Good when similar results can't be achieved with self-treatment. Boosts results of an at-home treatment program.

Deeper Resurfacing

The popularity of superficial peels and microdermabrasion is increasing, whereas the deeper peels and dermabrasion procedures we were doing ten years ago have declined significantly. That's a good thing. Not only is there a great deal of unpredictability with these deeper peels in terms of the results delivered but also dermabrasion is an aggressive and bloody procedure with an intense recovery period. While a few doctors may still be performing these deeper methods of resurfacing, on the whole they have gone by the wayside because of the more modern, less aggressive options such as Fraxel and lasers discussed in more detail below. If, however, you are planning a deeper resurfacing procedure, keep in mind that you will want to avoid going out in public for a week or even more, as your face will be very red, swollen, and oozy for several days and then crusty for a few more days after that.

"Don't jump when you hear about the latest and greatest laser. The media hype around the newest devices often precedes the safety testing. We have seen so many technologies come and go. A laser is not a magic wand, and worse, it may have undesirable consequences."

DR. KATHY FIELDS

Roll Baby, Roll

An alternative procedure for skin rejuvenation and treatment of acne scars that has been receiving more attention in the medical literature of late is micro-needling. This procedure is performed by rolling a device with approximately two hundred tiny needles that are 1.0mm to 2.0mm in length across the area of skin to be treated. The procedure, which requires local anesthesia, has been shown to trigger wound healing processes to produce new collagen fibers with results comparable to ablative techniques such as phenol peels, dermabrasion, and IPL lasers, but with less injury to the skin.[1]

Skin Rejuvenation Beams—Laser and Light Resurfacing

Skin rejuvenation beams include both lasers and multi-wavelength light technologies that stimulate collagen production and tighten the skin. A laser, which stands for light amplification by the stimulated emission of radiation, works by producing a single wavelength of light that is drawn to a particular color, delivering large amounts of energy to a small area. Lasers offer dermatologists a high level of precision and the ability to select a specific device for treatment of a specific concern.

We've found that when people hear the word "laser," expectations are heightened. It would be wonderful if lasers could act like a painless magic wand, performing miracles in one treatment. Unfortunately, this is not necessarily the case. While some lasers can be transformational, not all lasers are so miraculous and frequently involve some level of discomfort and the need for multiple treatments to achieve benefits. And it is important to understand that these devices wield a lot of power, meaning that if procedures are performed incorrectly, permanent damage can result. Therefore, it's crucial to select a highly skilled dermatologist who works with lasers all the time and to be realistic about what lasers do well and what issues they cannot successfully treat.

In general, lasers are excellent for treating skin texture, acne scars, isolated age spots, birthmarks, and hair removal. Vascular or pulsed dye lasers are outstanding for treating small blood vessels on the face but are not optimal for the tiny blood vessels on the legs, where the best method is injection sclerotherapy. Similarly, lasers are not the ideal treatment for hyperpigmentation and melasma. In fact, topical treatments are often more effective, less expensive, and have fewer potential side effects. And for sagging skin, the gold standard is still surgery and deep fillers, which we'll discuss a bit later in this and the next chapter.

"Several years ago, I embarked on a research study to evaluate the recovery rates associated with various wound treatments following deeper resurfacing procedures such as CO_2 lasers. Upon interviewing the study participants, I observed that, despite the informed consent, many of the women did not anticipate the phases of healing or the extensiveness of the recovery time. For most of the study participants, the results were quite impressive, but these are definitely not procedures for the faint-hearted."

LORI BUSH

⊕ This is How We Roll

Our interest in micro-needling led us to experiment with rollers containing shorter needles that do not penetrate to living cells. We conducted our own studies demonstrating that even superficial rolling can "trick" skin into behaving as if it has been wounded, leading to more abundant collagen production. We've found that by incorporating just a minute per day of rolling into a non-prescription skincare regimen, we can achieve impressive results for line and wrinkle reduction, pore tightening, and skin firming, all pain-free and without an appointment.[2]

Catch the Energy Wave

Thermage, a time tested radiofrequency device, and Ulthera, a newer ultrasonic procedure, use heat energy to tighten the skin. The heat penetrates more deeply than other lasers so that the top layer of the skin doesn't burn and there is no visible injury. Both work by stimulating the body's natural collagen production. The technology has recently improved, and risks of side effects have lessened. We are seeing tightening in our patients' skin. The cost has also come down, making them compelling therapies for those experiencing pronounced facial sagging.

Ablative versus Nonablative Lasers

Nonablative lasers work below the surface of the skin, treating without vaporizing the surface. The most commonly used group of lasers, they are widely used to reduce the appearance of blood vessels and brown spots. Although nonablative lasers leave no visible wound, redness, scaling, or welting of the skin can follow treatment. Overall, nonablative techniques carry fewer risks than ablative lasers, but many require multiple treatments to achieve desired results.

Rarely used anymore but worth mentioning, ablative lasers utilize carbon dioxide or erbium light sources to briefly direct an intense burst of laser energy onto the surface of the skin to treat severe skin aging and sun damage. They target water found inside the cells of the skin and vaporize it, along with the skin tissue, removing the entire top layer of the skin. This is basically a controlled burn with the many associated risks, including scarring, changes in pigment, and infection. The healing time is long, comparable to that for a face-lift. Although results are often dramatic, these procedures come at quite a price in terms of risk and recovery time. Unlike the fractionated ablative and fractionated nonablative lasers (see table below) that can be used to treat the neck, chest, and hands, only the face may be treated with the ablative lasers. Very few dermatologists are still using ablative lasers because of the safer options now available.

In the following table, we provide an overview and our ratings for the various options in laser and light therapy to give you a perspective on what each technology can and cannot do. Starting with the least aggressive therapy and moving to the most aggressive, we discuss what the treatment entails; the potential risks, discomfort, and downtime associated with each; and the cost and number of treatments needed.

Finally, we give an overall evaluation of each therapy. We will let you know whether we consider the treatment to be a YES (the technology is safe and effective) or a WATCH & WAIT (a technology that has not yet been proven and for which we recommend waiting a year or two to see whether it stands the test of time). We have not included any technology either that we deem too risky or that has a history of complications, side effects, or expense that is too great for the minimal improvement it delivers.

> "How do we know that some devices are not causing faster aging? Could they possibly be causing long-term damage that may not be apparent for several decades? In the 1960s X-ray therapy was a common treatment for severe facial acne, but thirty to forty years later it became evident that this treatment led to the development of skin cancers. That's why, for many of these laser treatments, a cautious 'wait and see' attitude is wise."
>
> **DR. KATIE RODAN**

Will Rejuvenation Treatments Make Cold Sores Flare?

If you have a history of herpes simplex virus (HSV) infections, including cold sores, shingles, or herpes, there is a high risk that laser resurfacing or filler treatment will cause a flare. To prevent the trigger of cold sores the tender cluster of tiny blisters around the mouth, oral antiviral treatments such as Acyclovir or Valtrex should be started prior to the rejuvenation procedure.

Light and Laser Resurfacing

TECHNOLOGY	TOUTED BENEFITS	TREATMENT	DOWNSIDE	RATING
LED (light-emitting diodes) i.e., *Gentlewaves Omnilux*	Improves tone, texture, and fine wrinkling. Painless and takes only a few minutes per treatment.	Low-energy light stimulates cellular energy. Weekly treatments for six weeks at approx. $100 per session.	Jury still out on efficacy other than for treatment of post chemical peel redness and inflammation. Some wavelengths may trigger other skin issues. Flashing lights have been reported to cause migraines or seizures.	WATCH & WAIT
IPL (intense pulsed light) i.e., *Palomar Starlux, Lumenis One, Ellipse IPL*	Reduces superficial brown spots, blood vessels, and facial redness associated with sun damage or rosacea. Pores, texture, and tone may also be subtly improved. Light energy is absorbed by the targeted tissue, leaving surrounding tissue intact.	Fifteen-minute sessions are spaced at four- to six-week intervals. Annual maintenance is required for some conditions. Cost is $300 to $600 per treatment.	Minor discomfort; oftentimes a topical anesthetic is applied prior to procedure. Swelling may occur but usually lasts only a few hours. Blistering rarely occurs but generally heals in about a week without scarring.	YES
PDL (pulsed dye laser) i.e., *Candela V Beam, Cynosure Vstar*	Extremely accurate laser that has stood the test of time. Excellent for large red blood vessels on the nose and cheeks; eliminates cherry angiomas (small red/purple spots on the body). Treats the redness of rosacea and many birthmarks.	Sessions take fifteen minutes and are spaced at four- to six-week intervals; two to three treatments are usually needed. With a condition such as rosacea, annual maintenance is advised. Cost is $150 for small spot, $600 for full face.	Possibility of burning and blistering of skin; bruising is likely and lasts for seven to ten days.	YES
ND: Yag Laser Candela i.e., *Gentle YAG, Cutera CoolGlide*	Effectively takes the pigment out of sun spots or brown spots.	Brown spot is numbed and then zapped with the laser. The area bruises and almost bleeds. Over five to seven days, the treated area sloughs off, and the spot disappears. If the color returns, additional treatments may be needed. Cost is $100 to $300 per treatment.	Minor discomfort, comparable to a rubber band snapping on your skin. Downtime is minimal, depending on the number of lesions treated. Small dell scarring (shallow indentations that make skin appear wavy) is rare but possible.	YES

TECHNOLOGY	TOUTED BENEFITS	TREATMENT	DOWNSIDE	RATING
Nonablative Fractionated Lasers i.e., *Fraxel Reliant, Fraxel Restore, Palomar 1540 Fractional, Cynosure 1440 nm Affirm*	Penetrates the dermis with discrete patterns of microscopic wounds to promote new collagen production and reduce wrinkles. Improves skin tone and texture, eliminating red matting on the neck and reducing the appearance of cobblestone skin.	Antiviral medicines are prescribed prior to treatment to prevent herpes outbreak. Topic anesthetic is applied. Treatment takes approximately thirty minutes; three to five treatments spaced a month apart are required. Benefits vary depending on power used, skin type, and healing response. May take several months following final treatment to see the full benefit. Cost is $1,000 to $1,500 per treatment.	Slightly to moderately painful. Mild sunburn sensation for an hour or two afterward. Swelling is minimal and generally resolves in a day or two. Skin remains pink for five to seven days following treatment. Eyes tend to swell. Because of possibility of significant peeling, patients often wait to return to work for four to five days. Because this treatment may provoke breakouts, acne-prone individuals are often prescribed a daily oral antibiotic.	YES
Fractionated Ablative CO_2 Lasers i.e., *Reliant Fraxel Repair, Lumenis Deep FX, Mixto, Sciton ProFractional*	Results comparable to nonablative fractionated laser after only one to two treatments. Reduced risk of scarring, permanent loss of pigmentation, and downtime less compared to more aggressive lasers.	Antiviral medicines prescribed prior to treatment to prevent herpes outbreak. Topical anesthetic prior to thirty-minute treatment procedure. Depth of treatment controlled to treat conditions on the surface of the skin such as pores and texture or deeper conditions such as acne scarring. Cost is approx. $2,000–$3,000 per treatment.	Obvious wounding of the skin with swelling, oozing, and pinpoint bleeding. Within a few days, the surface of the skin heals, with minor crusting and extensive peeling. Healing and downtime is seven to ten days. Because this treatment may provoke breakouts, acne-prone individuals are often prescribed a daily oral antibiotic.	YES Despite the risks and healing time, these lasers are becoming popular. The procedure is new and may have permanent side effects such as color loss over time.
CO_2 and Erbium Ablative Lasers	Can produce dramatic results, removing deep wrinkles and tightening the skin. Highly effective for treating acne scars, with approximately 50% improvement after just one treatment.	Performed under general anesthesia, in some cases doctors will do a CO_2 laser as an in-office procedure after the face has been anesthetized with a nerve block. Treatment takes approximately one hour and costs $5,000–$7,000 plus fees for operating room and anesthesia.	Procedure includes high risk of infection; requires diligent wound care; 30% chance that skin will become permanently lighter because of loss of pigmentation in the treated areas, creating a demarcation between the face and the neck. Scarring is possible. Moderate pain: skin looks and feels very raw, swollen, and tender for two to three weeks. Healing continues for several months, and redness and swelling doesn't disappear for three to six months or longer. There is a downtime of two to three weeks following the procedure.	YES This procedure is not for all skin types and may cause a permanent lightening of pigmentation in treated areas.

Compliance Is Important for Your Long-Term Appearance, Health, and Safety:

1. CALL YOUR DOCTOR IF SOMETHING APPEARS WRONG: If you have any procedure and notice tiny blisters on your face or any other reaction that wasn't thoroughly explained to you, call your doctor immediately to reduce the risk of scarring and infection.

2. AVOID THE SUN: Strict sun avoidance is imperative in order to maintain the results that you just paid for and to protect your vulnerable skin from hyperpigmentation.

3. COMMUNICATE YOUR CONDITIONS: There are a few conditions your doctor should be aware of when it comes to effective facial resurfacing. Any of these facial procedures can trigger a severe facial herpes outbreak in patients who have a history of herpes, and patients who are on Retin-A may also have sensitive skin that requires adjustments to treatments.

As we've described above, there are quite a few choices in advanced skin resurfacing and laser and light source treatments. Just remember, one laser may achieve better results than another depending upon the condition you are looking to correct. Therefore, your condition needs to be matched to the right laser—and the right doctor.

Plump Has Never Looked So Good: What Is Volume Replacement Anyway?

Most of us spend a good portion of our lives trying to fight off fat for our health and our looks. But when it comes to our faces, a little bit of fat in the right place is just what we need to counter the sagging, drooping, and wrinkling that often accompany aging. As you get older, those healthy round cheeks and full lips of youth start to wane. The skeleton, muscle, and fat diminish, the skin's surface thins, and the fat pad depletes. The more facial fat you lose, the more excess skin, wrinkles, and sagging you're likely to experience.

Fixing it sounds pretty simple; just put on a little weight and your face should fill out again. Unfortunately, it's not that easy. In terms of facial fat, it's all about location and distribution. You don't necessarily want a fuller face overall. Volume needs to be strategically replaced for more prominent, round cheeks and a smooth transition between your lower eyelid and your upper cheek. So, sadly, gobbling down an extra pint of Häagen-Dazs just won't do the trick. There are, however, a variety of nonsurgical dermatologic treatments available that can add back some of the volume that nature has taken away.

In the past, efforts to regain a more youthful appearance focused on pulling and lifting the skin, primarily through face-lifts. The issue of fat loss wasn't even addressed. However, with a face-lift, you may look tighter but not necessarily younger. There are many celebrity examples of sixty-year-old women who may be wrinkle free but certainly don't look young. Just look at Joan Rivers, who jokes openly about her face-lifts in GEICO insurance commercials. Further, because face-lifts are major surgery with associated risks and recovery times, they are not the right choice for many women.

Today, we're moving from an era of stretching and tightening skin to the modern approach of plumping it. By adding volume through fillers, you can change the shape of your face, achieving a more natural-appearing youthful balance.

Buyer Beware

Annabel had her lips injected with some permanent filler by a "doctor" in a hotel suite. He told her it was a new longer-lasting collagen, but it most definitely was not any form of collagen we know. She came to us with an upper lip that looked like an overstuffed sausage. Since it was permanent filler, unfortunately, there was not much we could do for her. The choices were either to live with it or to surgically remove the materials. Annabel learned the hard way not to experiment with dicey clinics and unknown fillers. Bottom line: no matter what procedure you are considering, always go to a reputable, experienced, board-certified dermatologist or plastic surgeon. Just because a doctor can "legally" use a needle on a person's face doesn't mean he or she should. Before you fall for a "Botox bargain," do your homework.

Volume Replacement: The Basics

Volumizing fillers are some of the best tools doctors have today for restoring a youthful appearance. In general, this treatment is intended for people over the age of forty. Around this time their facial fat begins to noticeably diminish, creating a gaunt or weathered look. The goal of all fillers is the same—to add volume back to the face. However, the specific substances injected and the facial concern each injectable addresses vary. Keep in mind that not every filling substance is right for all areas on a face, so as dermatologists, we rely on a variety of fillers.

Generally, thicker substances are best for treating deeper creases and recontouring areas such as cheek hollows and the jawline. Thinner substances work better on fine lines and superficial wrinkles or in areas where the skin is thin, such as around the eyelids and the lip lines. Some of the key areas we like to build up through these treatments are the temples, the tear trough (the hollows under the eyes that make you look tired and sad), sunken cheeks, and the area around the mouth and chin. Replacing volume in these areas gives an instant youthful lift. For example, filling the tear trough by gently injecting material right above the bone can serve as an alternative to a lower eyelid surgery.

> "I view fillers like a carpenter looks at materials to fill a damaged wall. Deeper fillers like fat or Sculptra provide basic framework and support. Medium fillers like Restylane or Juvéderm repair a moderately deep crevice. Use them in the right places and the face can be beautifully restored."
>
> **DR. KATIE RODAN**

Each product is also injected in a unique manner, and there is a tremendous amount of artistry involved in selecting the appropriate filler and determining the amount and the placement of the injection. The most skilled dermatologists are adept at using a wide variety of fillers and will approach an aging face with combined methods that can include laser, volumizing fillers, and muscle relaxers such as Botox, which we will cover later in this chapter. When it comes to volume replacement, we personally like patients to return two to three weeks after their initial treatment so we can check and refine as needed. We can't make a fifty-year-old look thirty again, but we can create a very natural look so that a fifty-year-old looks her best.

Temporary Fillers

FILLER	WHAT IS IT?	WHAT TO EXPECT	FINE PRINT
Hyaluronic Acid (HA) Particulate Gels i.e., *Restylane, Perlane, Juvéderm, Juvéderm Ultra Plus*	Temporary filler, clear viscous gels made from cross-linked sugar molecules that are found naturally in skin. Restylane is preferred for moderate wrinkles, Perlane for deeper wrinkles.	After the skin has been anaesthetized, soft, malleable gels are injected through a very small needle. HA works similarly to a sponge, drawing in water and expanding to provide volume to the face. It's often used to soften the nasolabial folds.	Treatments last six months to a year or longer. May need two treatments for optimal results at the start. Bruising and swelling at the injection site are the major side effects. Allergic reactions are rare but could occur and be serious. Cost is $500–$700 per syringe.
Poly-L-Lactic i.e., *Sculptra*	Longer-lasting temporary filler that is used for more generalized (rather than localized) treatments.	Plumps up the temple areas, builds cheeks, plumps the back of hands. Reverses the appearance of facial wasting.	Gradual results are achieved, so multiple treatments are generally necessary. Rarely results in nodules that can be avoided if treated areas are diligently massaged for five days following treatment. Three to five treatments may last two years. Cost is $1,000–$3,000 per session.
Autologous Fat Transfer	Rebalances fat from body stores to the face.	Used when large volume of filler is needed.	Technique is difficult to perfect and fat grafting may be variable from patient to patient. Costs $5,000–$8,000. Lasts one year in some, permanently in others.
Calcium Hydroxylapatite (CAHA) i.e., *Radiesse*	Soft, natural-feeling substance that is injected deeply into skin.	Fills nasolabial creases, marionette lines, cheeks. Plumps temples and chin and backs of the hands.	One treatment is often sufficient. Lasts about one year. For best results a second injection is performed approximately four weeks after the first. Cost is $650–$850 per syringe.

What's Your Filler Filled With?

There are two basic types of fillers: temporary (absorbable) and permanent (nonabsorbable). The former are gradually broken down by the body; the latter are not. Temporary fillers include hyaluronic acid and collagen—which last three months to a year—and longer-lasting substances such as Sculptra, Radiesse, and fat, which persist for one to two years. They all require ongoing treatments because as they are gradually degraded and reabsorbed into the skin, the treated area will eventually return to its original contour.

On the other hand, permanent and semipermanent fillers such as liquid silicone and a variety of hybrid fillers containing tiny particles suspended in a hyaluronic acid or a collagen base are meant to last forever. They are much more controversial as a category because of the risks surrounding them.

If you are exploring the possibility of fillers, the following table will provide the basics you'll need: what each filler does, what you can expect from a treatment, and what you should avoid. Once you are armed with this information, you should work with your dermatologist to find the best treatment for your specific needs.

How Long Is "Long Lasting"?

Results of rejuvenation treatments are not permanent. Because you will continue to age after you have your fillers, peels, laser treatments, or even a face-lift, you will need to maintain the results you have achieved. We cannot stop the clock; we can only move it back and/or slow it down. Therefore, if you choose to stop your treatments, aging will occur from that point forward. In case you are wondering, your aging process will not be accelerated by these treatments.

Isn't Longer Lasting Better?
Should I Consider a Permanent Filler?

We don't recommend permanent fillers such as silicone for healthy patients who are looking to restore a youthful appearance. The reality is that there have been few studies conducted on the long-term consequences of permanent fillers. And even though they may have FDA approval, we are not convinced that all permanent fillers are safe. Why? Because the face is dynamic and constantly changing over time, it is nearly impossible to remove permanent fillers once they have been injected. So if you no longer like the way the filler looks as your face naturally changes, there is no way to have it removed.

In general, permanent fillers are not a good choice. However, permanent fillers may be a viable option for certain medical conditions such as a cleft palette or acne scars. In these cases, it is imperative that a highly experienced physician performs the procedure because if the location is missed by a millimeter, it can cause additional disfigurement. If you are considering a permanent filler for one of these conditions, make sure you have done your homework and proceed with extreme caution.

> "If you didn't have Angelina Jolie lips during your youth, then don't try to achieve them when you're older. You'll end up looking like a caricature of yourself or like someone who entered the 'witness protection program.' Remember that artificial beauty doesn't count. You won't look beautiful if you don't look natural."
>
> **DR. KATIE RODAN**

Liquid Silicone: Permanent Filler

Medical-grade silicone is a liquid composed of manmade silica polymers that has been used to treat wrinkles and scars for decades. During this treatment, microdroplets of silicone are injected into the skin. The body then produces collagen to surround these microdroplets in an effort to contain the foreign material.

Think of it as an oyster, which contains a piece of sand around which a pearl develops. Using the microdroplet technique, treatments are repeated monthly to gradually build up the affected area. Silicone works well for cases of severe lipodystrophy, which is facial wasting caused by diseases such as HIV. It can also work well for certain types of facial scars. However, when improperly injected, silicone can cause permanent lumps that can only be removed surgically.

Getting Your Fill of Beauty

Injectable fillers are transforming the way doctors help patients preserve a natural-looking, youthful appearance. The cosmetic possibilities increase seemingly weekly as we continuously learn new information about the products, techniques, and long-term benefits of fillers. As cosmetic dermatologists, this is one of the most exciting and satisfying areas of our work because of the breadth of safe and efficacious treatments available. So, if you're thinking you may be looking for a little more than your at-home skincare can provide, you may want to discuss the possibility of fillers with your dermatologist.

Avoiding "the Botox Look"

We've all seen those women and men who take things to the extreme. Think Joan Rivers and Michael Jackson. The same is true of Botox treatments. When performed properly with the goal of creating a natural appearance, the results can be fantastic. But when overdone, the result can be an unnatural, almost frozen expression.

Our advice is to talk to your doctor to achieve a natural look. We like to use the least amount of toxin we need in order to get the job done. Like any cosmetic procedure, it is okay to take your time. Start with just one area, say, your forehead, to see how you like it before you allow your doctor to inject multiple areas such as your crow's-feet and lips. You can always come back for more.

"Marie, the wife of a psychiatrist, never tells her husband about her semiannual botulinum toxin injections. Whenever she gets close to her next appointment, her husband always asks, 'Honey, are you angry?' She isn't angry at all. Her Botox has worn off, and the wrinkles have returned. No longer used to seeing them, her husband is misreading her unconscious expression as disapproval. That's how Marie knows it's time to come in for a touch-up and reclaim control over what her face is communicating to others."

DR. KATHY FIELDS

Muscle Relaxer: How to Get Rid of Your Mean Vibe

Have you ever looked in the mirror and seen two parallel creases between your eyebrows right above your nose? These lines that appear as we age can make us look cross, angry, sad, or downright mean. It is truly amazing how erasing these folds can transform your face, changing your entire expression and making you look happier and more relaxed. It can also change the way people respond to you.

What Is Botox, and How Does It Work?

Botox is a botulinum toxin that originated nearly fifty years ago to medically treat crossed eyes, or strabismus. It is now prescribed for more than 150 varying medical conditions from vocal chord issues and neurological problems to muscular dystrophy and hyperhidrosis, or excessive sweating. Approved by the FDA for cosmetic treatment in 2002, today it is used to reduce wrinkles created by muscle contractions such as frown lines, crow's-feet, forehead lines, and lip lines. The results can be truly amazing.

Here's how it works: Botox is injected into the skin and then migrates to the nerve, preventing the transmission of a chemical called acetylcholine from the nerve to the muscle that it controls. Without this signal, the muscle cannot contract, the skin relaxes, and the wrinkle it caused begins to fade. Because only the nerves that control the muscle are affected and not the skin itself, the sensation for this area is unaffected, leaving the skin feeling normal. The results of Botox are not permanent because the nerves begin to sprout new connections to the muscle after about three months, causing the muscle once again to begin to contract.

Preparing for Botox Injections

These are the rules of the road we give our patients:

- Avoid aspirin, Advil, and herbal supplements such as garlic, ginseng, and ginkgo, which can cause your blood to thin, to reduce your risk of bruising.

- Don't come on an empty stomach because you may get light headed.

- Avoid having injections done during your menstrual cycle, as your body may be more sensitive to pain.

- Bring a concealer with you, just in case you get a slight bruise.

- Icing the area before and afterward can cut down on the sting of the needle and swelling.

- Apply your topical anesthetic cream on the way to your appointment.

- Don't have your first treatment on the day of a big event; leave at least one week for the full effect of Botox to take effect and any bruising to subside.

THE TREATMENT ITSELF

Although requiring expertise, the treatment itself is extremely quick and relatively painless. Typically, Botox injections take only about two minutes for a dermatologist to perform. Treatment of expression lines around the eyes, lips, or forehead involves several tiny injections in the region. To minimize any sting that may accompany the injections, we offer our patients a topical anesthetic prior to the procedure.

> "We think of Botox as the twenty-first century's version of penicillin because of the vast array of conditions it can safely and effectively treat."
>
> **DR. KATHY FIELDS**

It takes approximately five days for the full effect of treatment to be noticed, the goal of which is to give your face a relaxed and natural look while still allowing for expressive features. Initially, you will need to keep up with your treatments frequently, typically about every three to four months. If treatments are regularly maintained, moderately etched wrinkles will soften in older patients, and lines will be prevented from becoming fully and permanently formed in younger patients.

WHEN DO YOU START?

When the wrinkles remain after the expression has left your face or if people keep asking whether you are angry when you are not, it may be time to consider Botox. For a few this may occur in the mid- to late-twenties; for others it may happen in the thirties or forties. In today's youth-oriented world, it is no longer unusual to get started on an antiaging plan when you're still young.

Botox is a preventative as well as a corrective. Dr. Rodan's twenty-five-year-old assistant is already asking her about Botox. That doesn't mean we are urging all twenty-five-year-olds to run out and have their crow's-feet injected, but in some cases it makes sense to start early.

Botox is also very versatile. It is an ideal complement to microdermabrasions, lasers, and fillers. The results of lasers and peels will be better if there is less muscle movement in the facial areas during healing. This treatment can therefore be used to extend the duration and effectiveness of many other cosmetic treatments.

?DID YOU KNOW?

BOTOX IS APPROVED FOR THE TREATMENT OF MIGRAINE HEADACHES.[3]

Botox and Fillers: Perfect Together

Sometimes combining Botox with other fillers is the perfect solution. Here's why: botulinum toxin is injected into facial muscles to relax them, thereby smoothing lines and wrinkles caused by repetitive facial movements. By contrast, fillers are injected below a crease, wrinkle, scar, or depression in order to "fill" it in, smoothing the surface of the skin. Botulinum toxin works very well in combination with fillers. In the forehead, Botox is the first line of treatment for creases between the eyebrows. In some cases, however, the line is too deep for Botox alone and Restylane may be used to fill in the remaining crease. Another area where combination therapy is ideal is around the eyelids. We use Botox to soften the muscle activity that causes crow's-feet to form and Restylane to fill in the hollowness around the eyes. When done this way, the filler and the Botox seem to last longer.

CAN BOTOX HELP WITH DEPRESSION?

A 2006 pilot study conducted by Dr. Eric Finzi and published in the *Journal of Dermatologic Surgery* found that Botox may even cure severe depression.[4] In the study, Finzi found that nine of the ten depressed patients recovered from their symptoms after getting Botox injections between their eyebrows. This was nearly twice the success rate found from antidepressants. The theory, according to Finzi, is that Botox makes you stop scowling, which directly relieves the depression through biofeedback to the brain. In other words, if you don't physically frown, you feel happier. It has also been conjectured that when you frown, you seem forbidding to others. Therefore, the less you frown, the more positively others react to you. In turn, you feel less depressed.

> "Many patients are horrified with the thought of having a toxin injected into their faces. I assure them that it is a 'pretty' poison and it works so well they're going to wish it was permanent."
>
> **DR. KATIE RODAN**

HOW CAN YOU BE SURE BOTOX IS SAFE?

We know that "botulism" sounds scary to some people, but botulinum toxin is actually extremely safe as supported by long-term safety and efficacy studies. As we mentioned before, for decades it has been used safely in large doses (a hundredfold stronger than what we use in cosmetic dermatology) to treat all kinds of chronic medical conditions. It is so safe and effective that we consider it the cornerstone of cosmetic dermatology.

Like all cosmetic procedures, do your research. If every cosmetic physician in your city is charging $400 for Botox and one clinic is charging $99, be skeptical. If it sounds too good to be true, it probably is. But, as long as you go to a reputable dermatologist, Botox is one of the most satisfying treatments because it almost always does what it is supposed to do, making it the most consistent and reproducible treatment available. We think of it as the aspirin of dermatology, the wonder drug of this medical field, because it has so many different uses. Rewards are high; risks are low. As we say, a little Botox goes a long way in allowing you to age better.

Designing Your Future

Having great skin is a lifetime commitment. The foundation for beautiful skin starts at your sink with the right skincare. Cosmetic procedures can enhance your results - resurfacing initiates greater collagen production by your skin, fillers address loss of volume, and muscle relaxers take care of those weathering dynamic wrinkles. Through the right combination of procedures performed by a talented practitioner, restoration of critical aspects of youthful facial architecture can be restored. And with restoration of bright, full facial contours, supported by effective daily skincare, comes a sunnier relationship with the world around you and the recognition that you can look great well into your golden years.

Which Treatment Is Best for Which Concern?

Test your knowledge—it may come in handy someday.

1. Forehead furrows
_____ A. Lasers
_____ B. Botox
_____ C. Fillers

2. Smile lines
_____ A. Lasers
_____ B. Botox
_____ C. Fillers

3. Lipstick lines/wrinkles around your mouth
_____ A. Lasers
_____ B. Botox
_____ C. Fillers

4. Crow's-feet
_____ A. Lasers
_____ B. Botox
_____ C. Fillers

5. Fine, crepey wrinkling on cheeks
_____ A. Lasers
_____ B. Botox
_____ C. Fillers

6. Sagging, loss of volume in face
_____ A. Lasers
_____ B. Botox
_____ C. Fillers

Answers: 1. B; 2. C; 3. B and C; 4. B and sometimes C; 5. A; 6. C.

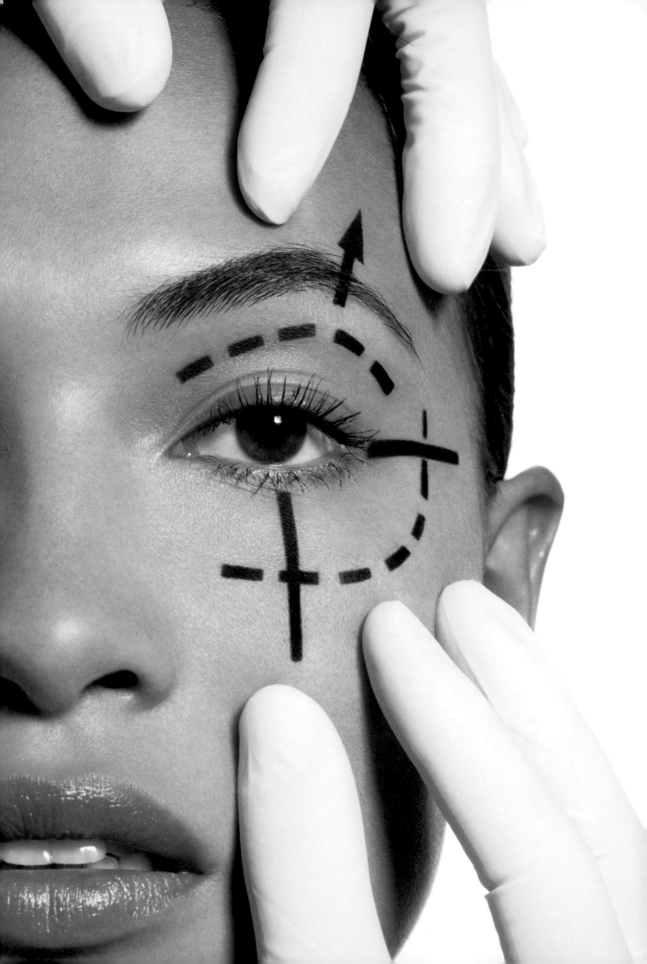

PLASTIC SURGERY

Is It Something I Should Consider?

"I can't remember a time when the changes in my skin became more obvious than when I looked down into a glass dresser top. It was then I saw my future, and I didn't like what I saw!"

Anonymous

We live in a youth-obsessed culture where beautiful women in their teens and twenties saturate the media. And who doesn't love to be told they look much younger than their years? It isn't surprising that there comes a time for many women and men when they start to wonder whether they are candidates for plastic surgery.

Is an "Extreme Makeover" in Your Future?

Reaching this threshold of discomfort with your looks can be a scary and emotional time. You may become distraught that the reflection in the mirror no longer resembles the image in your head. Or you may see young women on the street and wish you were them. Perhaps you even step back in time and hover over old photos or pull information about cosmetic procedures off the Internet. Yet, at the same time, you may feel guilty or shallow for even contemplating an expensive and risky solution to the natural process of getting older.

Today, the notion that cosmetic surgery can make life easier or better is not reserved just for the forty-five-plus set. Popular television features cosmetic surgery for everybody in shows such as *Doctor 90210*, *Extreme Makeover*, and *The Swan*.

In real life, however, it is only a very small percentage of the population that ever chooses elective surgery for aesthetic reasons. And while the majority of us think the appearance and health risks of face-lifts and eye surgery are "for other people, not me," more and more of us are considering taking the leap as we hope the means justify the physical and emotional ends.

If you are considering plastic surgery, we advise you to educate yourself about the procedures so you are fully prepared and realistic about the results each can deliver.

"If while stuck in traffic, you find yourself staring in the rearview mirror as you pull back your neck and face with your fingertips, wondering what you would look like with tighter skin, it may be time to consider cosmetic surgery. No cream in a jar is going to lift your skin back to where it used to be years ago."

DR. KATHY FIELDS

There's No Turning Back

Because these are precise and artistic surgeries and, unlike the options we discussed in the previous chapter, permanent, you will want to find the most reputable physician in the area. It's a good idea to get a referral from a friend who has had a similar procedure. Or, if your friends aren't talking, hairdressers often have the inside scoop from their clients and can offer great recommendations. Always consult with several plastic surgeons before you make your final decision. Look at before and after pictures of their work, talk with their staffs, and interview their patients. And because "beauty is in the eye of the beholder," make sure you find a surgeon whose goals are in sync with your own.

During your decision-making process, remember that many nonsurgical, preventive skincare choices are available to help you look your best. We encourage you to explore these noninvasive, low-risk options thoroughly before making a decision. Once you go under the knife to turn back the hands of time, there's no turning back.

Can Cosmetic Surgery Look Natural?

When performed by a talented surgeon, procedures such as face-lifts, midface-lifts, and blepharoplasty or eyelid surgery can look quite natural. However, cosmetic surgery is not a cure-all. If you long for a youthful appearance, your best approach is to protect and maintain your skin over your entire lifetime.

The human eye is so particular that a child can discern a one twenty-fifth-inch difference in the placement of an eyebrow.

Less is truly more for any procedure that may alter your appearance. Our faces are not perfectly symmetrical to begin with; eyes are usually a bit uneven, or one side of the face is often fuller than the other. Therefore, even working with a talented surgeon, you shouldn't expect to end up with a perfectly symmetrical face.

And remember that procedures such as face-lifts only pull skin up and across and don't replace lost volume, so you'll never look exactly as you once did. There is no way to look twenty-five when you're fifty. That's just not a realistic goal.

How Do I Know When I Need My Eyes Done?

Eyelid aging is hereditary, and some people are genetically predisposed to having hooded lids or bulging fat bags at an earlier age. In fact, it is not uncommon for a woman in her thirties to consider having her eyes done if she has some excess skin or fat deposits that make her look tired. For fatty, puffy eye bags the answer is almost always surgical removal or repositioning of excess fat or skin. We recommend that this be done early, before the lower lids are stretched to the point of no return and skin needs to be removed along with the fat. Removing skin is more risky in terms of lower lid droop; you don't want to end up looking like a basset hound. Keep in mind that removing skin may alter the shape of your eyes. If you wait to have a blepharoplasty when your upper lids are very droopy, the change will be more visible and thus harder to conceal but, in our opinion, still very much worth it.

> "When it comes to plastic surgery, timing is everything. Women who start too young with a face-lift in their early forties find themselves on a slippery slope. In order to maintain that firm 'youthful' face, they'll need a redo face-lift in their mid fifties and another one in their late sixties, eventually ending up with that scary 'wind-tunnel look.' Better to put up with a few wrinkles and wait a little longer. As for when the optimal time for plastic surgery is, I tell my patients that a loose, saggy turkey neck is their best indicator."
>
> **DR. KATIE RODAN**

What about My Sagging Neck?

Nora Ephron's book *I Feel Bad about My Neck* may echo the sentiments of many women as they enter their forties and fifties. Nothing gives away true age like a neck waddle.

There are three common signs of an aging neck:

- *Early neck aging manifests as two parallel bands running from the base of the chin to the sternum. These bands are caused by the thickening of the neck muscle called the platysma and respond beautifully to Botox injections.*

- *As aging advances, several prominent neck bands may appear. Because large amounts of Botox would be required to relax all of these platysmal bands, surgery is a far better option. Since there is no surgical procedure limited to the neck only, a true neck lift is in actuality a midface-lift, which will also pick up droopy jowls. We are hopeful that one day lasers and other radiofrequency treatments will be the answer to a saggy neck; however, we have not seen great results thus far.*

- *The third reason why someone might feel "bad about [his or her] neck" is the sagging and loss of the defined jawline caused by excess fat, or, in other words, a double chin. A simple, in-office liposuction procedure that removes excess fat can be quite successful and rewarding.*

When Should I Have a Face-Lift?

Today, women are having smaller surgical and injectable procedures such as neck liposuction and Restylane injections at younger ages to delay the need for more drastic work later on. As you age, you can make small, subtle changes that allow you to stay on top of the aging process. We want to dispel the idea that there is nothing you can do to help your skin yourself so that when it starts to hang, the only option is to head to the surgeon. We believe that it is better to preserve what you have for as long as you can and to save surgery as the last resort for when you really feel you need it.

With that said, we recommend a face-lift when you are unhappy with your sagging neck and jowls. Remember that there are some incredible nonsurgical fillers that do wonders to crisp up the jowl line (see Chapter Sixteen), so talk to your dermatologist about those options first. But once jowls and neck skin are significantly sagging, nothing is going to pick them back up except surgery.

There is no ideal age for a face-lift, and it varies from person to person. The trigger event is different for everyone and may be earlier than you think, with women opting for their first face-lift younger than in the past. In fact, the average age today is between forty-seven and fifty-five.

It is important to understand what a face-lift can and cannot do. For example, it does not treat lines and wrinkles, and it does not really address volume loss, unless fat transfer is done at the time of the surgery. Dermal fillers such as Restylane and Juvéderm can fine-tune the surgical results. That means a face-lift is part of the continuum of antiaging treatments. It addresses skin laxity by removing excess skin, tightening the loose muscles underneath, and elevating sagging soft tissue.

What Is Recovery Like?

If you opt for plastic surgery, make sure you are prepared for the prolonged healing time involved. Even in the easiest of cases, expect swelling and distortion for two to four weeks postoperatively and allow several months for your face to settle down entirely. Because of this extended downtime, you won't want to race back to work. In fact, if you have the opportunity, you should lay low for a month or so and then reenter the world with your new look.

During this healing phase, be on the lookout for real risks such as infection, asymmetry, or nerve damage. Should any of these occur, contact your physician immediately.

How Long Do These Cosmetic Surgery Procedures Last?

Unfortunately, improvements in the contours of the eyelids, face, and brows after skin tightening procedures are still subject to the continued effects of aging, gravity, and sun damage, with the results lasting around seven years. But the improvements can sometimes turn the clock back ten to fifteen years, so you will always look younger than your peers who have not undergone cosmetic procedures. And, if the surgery is performed well, you will certainly look younger than you would have if you had not had the procedure.

The Best Surgeons May Say "No"

Well-trained, ethical plastic surgeons are very conscientious about not performing a procedure if they believe the patient has unrealistic expectations or expects the procedure itself to fix an unhappy life. They will always be on the lookout for a psychological disturbance called body dysmorphic disorder. In these cases, which are estimated to affect as much as 1%–2% of the population, there is an intense preoccupation or obsession with one's own appearance. Even the smallest imperfections that are unnoticeable to others become sources of great angst or depression. This condition often starts in adolescence, affects males and females equally, and is often associated with other signs of obsessive-compulsive behavior. It is important to recognize and treat this disease because the incidence of suicide is almost double that of major depression. In cases such as these, cosmetic surgery is not the answer; psychiatric treatment is.

The sad truth is that you can always find a surgeon who is willing to do a procedure. But if you have to look too hard, that may be your first clue that something else needs professional care first.

Cosmetic Surgery or Not?

It takes courage to grow old, and the way in which you embrace it is an individual choice. The decision about cosmetic surgery is very personal and depends upon where you are in your life and how you want to approach the future. It's definitely not for everyone, but if it is a choice you wish to pursue, we want to encourage you to do your homework, talk to lots of friends and professionals beforehand, and make sure to find a surgeon you can trust. When done properly, the results can give you a whole new lease on life.

⮞ How Do You Find the Right Plastic Surgeon?

Here are some factors to consider:

1. Is the surgeon board certified by the American Board of Plastic Surgery? _____
Is the surgeon experienced?_____

Surgeons should have at least six years of training in plastic surgery and general surgery, with at least three years minimum in plastic surgery.

Consider how long the surgeon has been in practice. You should generally look for a physician with at least five years of experience.

2. Does the surgeon operate only in accredited medical facilities such as surgery centers and hospitals? _____

If the surgeon operates in office, the office must be accredited.

You can ask the receptionist about the facilities or do your own research on the World Wide Web. A great place to start is with the Better Business Bureau.

3. Does the surgeon specialize in your area of interest? _____

I.e., breast augmentation, facials, nose jobs, etc.

4. Do you like this individual's work? _____

Make sure to check out before and after pictures. There should be some on the office's Website or available for you to view in the office.

If the plastic surgeon doesn't meet all of these requirements, keep looking.[1]

Postscript: How We Came to Practice Dermatology

L ife takes you on a journey. Sometimes the journey is the one you planned. Sometimes it's to a place you never imagined. But if you believe in your dream, keep your eyes on the horizon, persevere even when the road gets bumpy, and, most important, work, work, and then work some more, you can reach further than you ever thought possible. We're proof of that. Nearly twenty-five years after we first met during our residencies at Stanford University School of Medicine, we continue to be passionate about every aspect of our careers. As practicing dermatologists, entrepreneurs, and skincare developers, we can't wait to get up in the morning and begin our next project, whether it's seeing a patient, creating a new skincare formulation, or talking to women about their skin issues. Our goal is to help empower both women and men to change their skin and their lives. We love the path we have created, and we continue to enjoy every moment of the journey.

Although it often feels like we've been on parallel paths forever—sometimes even our parents get us mixed up—the personal stories that brought us each to medical school in the first place are quite different.

Kathy's Story

My three siblings and I were destined to become physicians from birth. Not because we come from a family of doctors (my dad is an optometrist) but because our hardworking parents gave us the message that the most important and noble work we could pursue was to heal others by going into medicine. They would always point out our family friend, Dr. Ann, as a woman to emulate.

When I was twelve years old, we'd walk the Florida beaches with this ninety-year-old physician, and people would constantly stop to ask her all kinds of health questions. "See?" my dad would say. "Her work is really valued. She loves what she does, and she can keep doing it forever—no one can ever take it away."

They instilled in me, my twin brother, older sister, and younger brother the belief that we each needed to build a future that would grant us total financial independence. "You don't ever want to rely on anyone else," my mom and dad would say. I consider myself extremely fortunate that they shared this progressive message with their daughters forty years ago, when careers for women were far from the norm. They let us know that if we set a goal and worked our hardest, we could achieve anything.

But they didn't just give us this advice; they helped us navigate the difficult road to adulthood. In fact, they took on the role of career counselors, continually helping us strategize the best way to reach our goals. Without their patient guidance, we probably would have ended up like so many other high school kids, overwhelmed by the infinite number of career choices and even paralyzed when it came to making a decision. Instead, I was able to take charge and define my career rather than stumble into it.

I went to college in the late 1970s, when only about 10% of medical students were women. Getting into medical school was insanely competitive, and being a female was only a small advantage. It was a lot of work and a lot of pressure because I was competing with hundreds of other students in the same classes with the same goal, all fighting for the five top grades. Although I may not have been the life of the party back then, I was intensely determined, so I learned how to prioritize, eliminate distractions, and get the A.

After graduating from the University of Florida with a BS in neurobiochemistry, I attended medical school at the University of Miami in Florida with my twin brother, Ken. After four years of college, starting eight more years of school seemed daunting. But because I had my twin, who also happened to be my best friend, by my side day in and day out, medical school was not only doable but also fun. Together, we attacked every problem head-on. We took the attitude that no matter how gross, difficult, or potentially uninteresting a course or rotation was, we would "go positive" and find the relevance or value in it. In fact, we quickly learned that if we wasted time whining, things only got harder academically and we didn't win any friends along the way. This "go positive" mantra helped get us through the tough times and is still what I say to my kids when they are frustrated by a challenge.

After graduating from medical school, I became an obstetrics/gynecology intern. I loved delivering babies, performing surgery, and working with women. However, I discovered that I fainted when surgeries went over three hours (I couldn't physically stay on my feet in one place for that long). This made me question whether ob was the ideal specialty for me.

One day my mother suggested I look into dermatology, which I had never before considered because I thought it might be "wimpy." Boy, was I wrong. As I investigated it more, I discovered it was exciting, challenging, and a perfect fit for me. Before I committed to dermatology, however, I participated in a fungal study in the jungles of Columbia. That was a crazy, risky adventure filled with the Columbian army, threats from drug lords, and lots of poisonous creepy crawlies. But I survived, and never again did I use the words "wimpy" and "dermatology" in the same breath. From then on, I was sold on skin and was accepted into the dermatology residency program at Stanford University.

Although medical school and residency involved eight years of very hard work with insane hours and rarely a weekend off, to this day I'm thrilled with my career choice. I've never once been bored, and I get to work with children, teens, men, and women, from pediatrics to geriatrics. There is plenty of surgery, fabulous cosmetic procedures that let me be creative, and a good amount of time home with my family.

As for the rest of the Fields clan—yup, they're all happily practicing medicine. My wonderful twin brother, Ken, is a dermatologist, too. My big sister, Connie, is a cardiologist, and my little brother, Dan, is an ER doc. I respect them greatly. They wear many halos and are true heroes because they save lives every day. We call each other many times a week and have loads to share. We are all delighted with our career choices. Seems that mom and dad knew us well.

As a mother myself, the message I hope I can pass on to my two sons is that you must find your passion, learn what it takes to turn that into a productive career, and commit yourself to doing what it takes to get there. And, importantly, I hope my sons will relish the journey, because every day is a gift to be celebrated.

Katie's Story

Unlike Kathy, I never dreamed of becoming a doctor when I was growing up. Every relative of mine is either a lawyer or a judge, so a career in law seemed to be my familial destiny. In fact, as a history major, that was the direction I was heading in until my junior year, when I took a business law class. I was bored out of my mind and got the worst grade of my college experience. I realized then that I needed to reevaluate my future.

Fortuitously, that summer my cousin recommended me for a job at a cardiovascular research lab at a major Los Angeles hospital. She was leaving the position and convinced me that it would be more interesting and better paying than the waitressing job I had lined up. I thought, "Why not?"

On the first day, the lab director gave me and the other summer interns—two premed students from Stanford, a medical student from UCLA, and Linda, a recent graduate from the USC English department—a tour of the lab. Showing us a diagram of the circulatory system, he described the anatomy of the heart. I was enthralled. Since my only science classes in college were "Football Physics" and "Rocks for Jocks," i.e., easy classes that fulfilled graduation requirements, I had no clue as to the inner workings of the body. From that day on, I discovered a whole new world of science and medicine.

One day during lunch, Linda told me that following her internship at the lab, she was applying to medical school. Because she didn't fit the stereotype of the nerdy guy with the biochemistry major, the look of shock must have been written all over my face.

"As a matter of fact," she added, "even you could do it. All you need are four science courses to qualify for medical school."

No one had ever before suggested there was even a remote possibility I could become a doctor. Little did Linda know what a turning point our conversation was for me. Upon returning to the University of Virginia for my final year, I immediately met with the premed advisor. Believe it or not, he didn't call me delusional for wanting to be a doctor even after he heard that, since high school, I hadn't taken a real science or math class. Instead, he confirmed what Linda had told me: med school entry required two years of chemistry and one year each of biology and physics. While I could cram all of these courses into a single very intense year, he wisely suggested I finish my history degree first, just in case.

My parents, on the other hand, dropped the phone after I told them about my new, exciting plans. Talk about a potential confidence crusher when the two people who know you better than anyone else in the world bluntly tell you, "Yes, you are delusional!" Fortunately, my gut told me not to listen, and I went full speed ahead.

As predicted, the next year was intense. The premed courses were difficult, and my classmates were competitive beyond anything I had ever before experienced. Believing I had to get all As to prove that a girl with a BA in history really could hack medical school, I put myself under immense pressure. As if that weren't enough, I had to score high on the MCATs (medical school entry exams) just to get in. I might as well have joined the Marine Corps (that would have made my dad really happy), because I was surely in academic boot camp.

The MCAT was an experience I will never forget. I felt good about the test until the last section before the lunch break. When the buzzer sounded, I still had a third of the section to finish. Feeling like I'd flunked the test and that my dream was over, I called home. Between my sobs, my parents gave me the following excellent advice; "Wash your face, eat your lunch, and phone us back." As they so wisely knew, I wouldn't be making that call because I hate to quit. I went back to finish the afternoon portion of the test, and my hard work and perseverance paid off: my test scores and science grades passed muster with the admissions committee.

My med school class of 1983 was composed of mostly male hard-core science majors who were genetically programmed to be doctors. I discovered what an anomaly I was and how my in-depth knowledge of the Doctrine of Manifest Destiny didn't help me much when it came to memorizing the Krebs cycle. My fear of failure often got the better of me, causing me to lie awake in bed at night fretting over whether the school had made a mistake accepting me and wondering whether I would even graduate.

Noticing my exhaustion, my faculty advisor said, "Instead of worrying, do something worthwhile like getting out of bed and studying." Sounds pretty simple, but it was one of the best pieces of advice I've ever received. From then on, I replaced worry with work, a far more productive way of channeling my anxiety.

After successfully completing that first year, school became easier. With each small success, my self-esteem and confidence grew. Before long, I was the happiest med school student and intern on campus. I knew my decision to enter medicine was right, and I was grateful for the opportunity.

From day one of medical school, I knew dermatology was my calling. Like most teenagers, I'd had my acne woes. Indeed, I had been obsessed with my skin. Each and every pimple seemed to chip away at my self-esteem. I was the girl who wanted to stay home from school because of her breakouts, the one who ripped up her eleventh-grade photo because she hated the way she looked. I tried every prescription and concocted every home remedy I discovered in books and magazines. Because of my firsthand experience, I knew that as a doctor I could identify with dermatology patients. I understood that skin disease is more than skin deep and that it affects not only the way the world sees you, but also how you see yourself.

As it turns out, it was a match made in heaven. I followed my passion, never looking back or regretting my decision, and I've never been bored a single day of my career. My mantra is, "It isn't work if you love what you do." As the mother of two daughters, I hope my circuitous career path has taught them the value of having lots of life experiences without preconceived notions of where those experiences might take them. I also hope they have seen that nothing worthwhile ever comes easily. Just because you have a dream doesn't mean that getting there will be a smooth ride. When they hit the "speed bumps," I give them their grandparents' advice: wash your face, eat your lunch, and remember why you're driving down this road in the first place. With every obstacle they surmount, their confidence and self-esteem will grow and bring their dreams one step closer to reality.

Diving into the Business World

After we completed our residencies at Stanford, we each started our own individual dermatology practices in the San Francisco area and discovered there were a lot of people whose everyday skincare concerns were not being met. The lack of effective over-the-counter and prescription treatments created frustration and a sense of hopelessness for our patients. This was an "aha" moment for both of us. We saw a need to develop skincare products based on medicines that could treat everyone effectively and affordably.

At the time, we had no idea what this would mean. We never thought we'd end up running a business while continuing to practice medicine, but developing products became a labor of love. By following our passion, we blindly became businesswomen and entrepreneurs. Once again, the learning curve was huge, long, and hard. We had more than a few setbacks and made lots of mistakes along the way, but thankfully, we had each other to lean on when we started to feel discouraged.

Our hard work and commitment have been worthwhile. Through our medicated skincare solutions, we have been able to help millions of people. This book is a continuation of our desire to help each of you achieve a healthy and beautiful complexion. We hope we've helped you realize that taking care of your skin does not need to be difficult or expensive. Remember that by setting a goal, educating yourself about the issue at hand, and being proactive about your future, you really can change your skin and change your life.

Bibliography

INTRODUCTION HOW VANITY CAN HELP YOU GO THE DISTANCE

1. Etcoff, Nancy. 1999. *Survival of the Prettiest: The Science of Beauty*. New York: Doubleday.

2. Jablonski, Nina J. 2006. *Skin: A Natural History*. Berkeley: University of California Press.

3. Morris, Desmond. 2005. *The Naked Woman: A Study of the Female Body*. New York: Thomas Dunne Books, an imprint of St. Martin's Press.

CHAPTER 1 YOUR SKIN'S DESTINY

1. Cherkas, Lynn F., Janice L. Hunkin, Bernet S. Kato, J. Brent Richards, Jeffrey P. Gardner, Gabriela L. Surdulescu, Masayuki Kimura, Xiaobin Lu, Tim D. Spector, and Abraham Aviv, MD. 2008. "The association between physical activity in leisure time and leukocyte telomere length." *Archives of Internal Medicine* 168, no. 2. http://archinte .ama-assn.org/cgi/content/full/168/2/154?maxtoshow=&HITS=10&hits=10&RESUL TFORMAT=&fulltext=Kings+College+2008+twins&searchid=1&FIRSTINDEX =0&resourcetype=HWCIT.

CHAPTER 2 SKINCARE TRUTHS AND MYTHS

1. Benson, Linda R. 2000. "New research finds smoking, wrinkles battle at molecular level." Review of John Zone's 1996 study, by John Zone. *Dermatology Times*, (Sep.1): 40.

2. Kings College London: University of London. June 14, 2005. "Smoking and Obesity Accelerate Human Ageing."

3. Schmich, Mary. 1997. "Advice, like youth, probably just wasted on the young." *Chicago Tribune*, June 1, Metro Chicago section.

4. National Sleep Foundation. 2008. http://www.sleepfoundation.org/sites/default/ files/2008%20POLL%20SOF.PDF

5. Stegman, Samuel J., MD. 1987. "Sleep creases." *American Journal of Cosmetic Surgery* 4: 277–280.

6. Chiu, Annie, Susan Y. Chon, and Alexa B. Kimball. 2003. "The response of skin disease to stress." *Archives of Dermatology* 139: 897–900.

7. Carol, Ruth. "Rosy cheeks could be rosacea." *Dermatology Insights* 3, no. 1: 23.

8. Park, Madison. "Advice to Obama on battling presidential aging." CNNhealth.com. http://www.cnn.com/2009/HEALTH/01/06/presidential.health.aging/index.html.

CHAPTER 3 HURRICANE OF HORMONES

1. Brizendine, Louann, MD. 2006. *The Female Brain*. New York: Doubleday Broadway Publishing Group.

2. Steingraber, Sandra, PHD. 2007. "The falling age of puberty: A breast cancer fund report." San Francisco: Breast Cancer Fund.

3. Stolla, Steven, Alan R. Shalita, Guy F. Webster, Richard Kaplan, Sid Danesh, and Alyson Penstein. 2001. "The effect of the menstrual cycle on acne." *Journal of the American Academy of Dermatology* 45: 957–960.

4. Lucky, Anne W., Frank M. Biro, Loretta A. Simbartl, John A. Morrison, and Nancy W. Sorg. 1997. "Predictors of severity of acne vulgaris in young adolescent girls: Results of a five-year longitudinal study." *Journal of Pediatrics* 130, issue 1: 30–39.

5. Lucky, Anne W. 2004. "Quantitative documentation of a premenstrual flare of facial acne in adult women." *Archives of Dermatology* 140: 423–424.

6. "Bone health and osteoporosis." October 14, 2004. A Report of the Surgeon General. Washington, DC: Office of Public Health and Sciences, United States Department of Health and Human Services.

7. Rigotti, N. A., R. M. Neer, S. J. Skates, D. B. Herzog, and S. R. Nussbaum. 1991. "The clinical course of osteoporosis in anorexia nervosa: A longitudinal study of cortical bone mass." *Journal of the American Medical Association* 265, no. 9 (March 6), http://jama.ama-assn.org/cgi/content/abstract/265/9/1133.

8. WebMD. "Depression in women." http://www.webmd.com/depression/guide/depression-women.

9. Chlebowski, Rowan T., Susan L. Hendrix, Robert D. Langer, Marcia L. Stefanick, Margery Gass, Dorothy Lane, Rebecca J. Rodabough, Mary Ann Gilligan, Michele G. Cyr, Cynthia A. Thomson, Janardan Khandekar, Helen Petrovitch, and Anne McTiernan. 2003. "Influence of estrogen plus progestin on breast cancer and mammography in healthy postmenopausal women." *Journal of the American Medical Association* 289, no. 24 (June 25): 3243–3253.

10. Guyuron, Bahman. 2007. Kiehn-Desprez Professor and Chair. Department of Plastic Surgery. University Hospitals of Cleveland and Case Western Reserve University.

CHAPTER 5 HERE COMES THE SUN

1. National Cancer Institute. 2007. "Cancer trends progress report: 2007 update." http://progressreport.cancer.gov.

2. Feldman, S. R., A. Liguori, M. Kucenic, S. R. Rapp, A. B. Fleischer, W. Lang, and M. Kaur. 2004. "Ultraviolet exposure is a reinforcing stimulus in frequent indoor tanners." *Journal of the American Academy of Dermatology* 51: 45–51.

3. The Skin Cancer Foundation. 2008. "Skin cancer facts." http://www.skincancer.org/Skin-Cancer-Facts/.

4. Linos, Eleni, Susan M. Swetter, Myles G. Cockburn, Graham A. Colditz, and Christina A. Clarke. 2009. "Increasing burden of melanoma in the United States." *Journal of Investigative Dermatology* 129, no. 7: 1666–1674.

5. International Agency for Research on Cancer, special report on radiation, *Lancet*, August 2009, online edition.

6. Russak, JE, Rigel, DS. 2010. "Tanning bed hygiene: microbes found on tanning beds present a potential health risk." *Journal of the American Academy of Dermatology* 62, issue 1: 155-157.

7. American Academy of Dermatology. *Skin Cancer Self-Examination Shower Card.*

CHAPTER 6 RAISE YOUR EXPECTATIONS

1. U.S. Food and Drug Administration. July 8, 2002; updated April 30, 2012. "Is it a cosmetic? A drug? Or both?" http://www.fda.gov/Cosmetics/GuidanceComplianceRegulatoryInformation/ucm074201.htm?utm_campaign=Google2&utm_source=fdaSearch&utm_medium=website&utm_term=is%20it%20a%20cosmetic?%20a%20drug?%20or%20both?

CHAPTER 7 VISITING A DERMATOLOGIST

1. Tay, Angela. 2009. "Top wedding day worries of brides revealed!" Ezine Articles. http://ezinearticles.com/?Top-Wedding-Day-Worries-Of-Brides-Revealed!&id=1207089.

CHAPTER 8 ACNE AND ROSACEA

1. American Academy of Dermatology. 2009. *Acne.* http://www.aad.org/media/background/factsheets/fact_acne.html.

2. Cordain, Loren, Staffan Lindeberg, Magdalena Hurtado, Kim Hill, S. Boyd Eaton, and Jennie Brand-Miller. 2002. "Acne vulgaris: a disease of western civilization." *Archives of Dermatology* 138: 1584–1590.

3. Smith, Robyn N., Neil J. Mann, Anna Braue, Henna Mäkeläinen, and George A. Varigos. 2007. "A low-glycemic-load diet improves symptoms in acne vulgaris patients: a randomized controlled trial." *American Journal of Clinical Nutrition* 86, no. 1: 107–115.

4. Adebamowo, Clement A., Donna Spiegelman, F. William Danby, A. Lindsay Frazier, Walter C. Willett, and Michelle D. Holmes. 2005. "High school dietary dairy intake and teenage acne." *Journal of the American Academy of Dermatology* 52, issue 2: 207–214.

5. American Academy of Dermatology. 1997. *Acne and American Teens Survey.*

6. Jancin, Bruce. 2004. "Teens with acne cite shame, embarrassment about skin." *Skin and Allergy News* 35:28.

7. AMP Insights, research division of Alloy Inc. 2003. "Lose the zits" survey.

8. Ozolins, Mara, and E. Anne Eady, Anthony J. Avery, William J. Cunliffe, Alain Li Wan Po, Ciaran O'Neill, Nick B. Simpson, Christina E. Walters, Ellen Carnegie, Jennifer B. Lewis, John Dada, Mary Haynes, Karen Williams, and Hywel C. Williams. 2004. "Comparison of five antimicrobial regimens for treatment of mild to moderate inflammatory facial acne vulgaris in the community." *The Lancet* 364, issue 9452: 2188–2195.

9. National Rosacea Society. "What is rosacea?" Rosacea.org. http://www.rosacea.org/index.php.

10. K.Rodan, K. Fields, L.Bush, L.Zhang and T.Falla. "Down-regulation of cathelicidin activity for management of rosacea-related symptoms and hyperirritable skin." 68th American Academy of Dermatology Meeting. February 2011. New Orleans, LA.

11. Tan, Stephen R., and Whitney D. Tope. 2004. "Pulsed dye laser treatment of rosacea improves erythema, symptomatology, and quality of life." *Journal of the American Academy of Dermatology* 51, issue 4: 592–599.

CHAPTER 9 SKIN DISCOLORATIONS

1. Fink, Bernhard, Karl Grammer, and Paul J. Matts. 2006. "Visible skin color distribution plays a role in the perception of age, attractiveness, and health in female faces." *Journal of Evolution and Human Behavior* 27: 433–442.

2. Unpublished data, Rodan + Fields, July - August, 2012.

CHAPTER 10 RED/SENSITIVE SKIN

1. Garg, Amit, Mary-Margaret Chren, Laura P. Sands, Mary S. Matsui, Kenneth D. Marenus, Kenneth R. Feingold, and Peter M. Elias. 2001. "Psychological stress perturbs epidermal permeability barrier homeostasis: Implications for the pathogenesis of stress-associated skin disorders." *Archives of Dermatology* 137: 53–59.

2. Robles, Theodore F. 2007. "Stress, social support, and delayed skin barrier recovery." *American Psychosomatic Society* 69, no. 8: 807–815.

CHAPTER 16 INTERVENTION

1. Majid, Imran. 2009. "Microneedling Therapy in Atrophic Facial Scars: An Objective Assessment." *Journal of Cutaneous and Aesthetic Surgery* 2, issue 1: 26-30.

2. Unpublished data, Rodan + Fields, June, 2011.

3. U.S. Food and Drug Administration. 2010. "FDA approves Botox to treat chronic migraine." http://www.fda.gov/NewsEvents/Newsroom/PressAnnouncements/ucm229782.htm.

4. Finzi, Eric, and Erika Wasserman. 2006. "Treatment of depression with botulinum toxin a: A case series." *American Society for Dermatologic Surgery* 32: 645–650.

CHAPTER 17 PLASTIC SURGERY

1. American Society of Plastic Surgeons. ASPS Member Qualifications. http://www.plasticsurgery.org/Articles-and-Galleries/Patient-and-Consumer-Information/ASPS-Member-Qualifications.html

Index

Acknowledgments

Our love and gratitude go out to an extraordinary team of colleagues, friends, and family who passionately "lived the book" with us. The crazy long hours of editing, fact-checking, referencing, and design debates certainly stressed psyches and skin. Thankfully, a little extra exfoliation, meditation, and plenty of sunscreen should have everybody back to radiant, glowing, and rational by time of publication.

From the inception of the concept to the finished manuscript, Mimi Field and Hilary Martin worked closely with us, offering invaluable input and energetically helping us craft and recraft every single word. Mimi even shared her beautiful baby with us when it was time for the photo session.

With a brilliant eye, Courtney Winget offered her thoughtful edits on the manuscript and book design, flying back and forth from Utah to San Francisco on a weekly basis. And even more important, with grace and good humor, she kept us on a tight schedule to ensure that this book actually became a reality.

Katie's daughter, Elana Rodan, supplied a fresh eye with her careful reading, in-depth research, and thoughtful comments. Even though she comes at it from a different discipline, she clearly shares her mom's vision of great skin for all.

Our heartfelt thanks to Christian Hansen and his team at Hint® Creative for their superb design guidance and to the team at the Jenkins Group for literally putting the words to paper.

And to Amnon, Erin, Mary, Lindsay, Nancy, Jade, Garry, Richie, Mark, Daniela, Steve, and Zack: thanks for tolerating us when we were at our most intolerable.

Finally, this book could not exist without our patients and the other women in our lives who continually inspire us to stay in the game. Their personal life experiences have enriched our lives and the pages of this book.